Hormone Balance for Women

An Easy Program to Master Metabolism, Detox Body, Keep Fit, Boost Energy and Live younger

HATTIE ELLEDGE

The content contained within this book may not be reproduced, duplicated or transmitted without direct written permission from the author or the publisher.

Under no circumstances will any blame or legal responsibility be held against the publisher, or author, for any damages, reparation, or monetary loss due to the information contained within this book. Either directly or indirectly.

Legal Notice:

This book is copyright protected. This book is only for personal use. You cannot amend, distribute, sell, use, quote or paraphrase any part, or the content within this book, without the consent of the author or publisher.

Disclaimer Notice:

Please note the information contained within this document is for educational and entertainment purposes only. All effort has been executed to present accurate, up to date, and reliable, complete information. No warranties of any kind are declared or implied. Readers acknowledge that the author is not engaging in the rendering of legal, financial, medical or professional advice. The content within this book has been derived from various sources. Please consult a licensed professional before attempting any techniques outlined in this book.

By reading this document, the reader agrees that under no circumstances is the author responsible for any losses, direct or indirect, which are incurred as a result of the use of the information contained within this document, including, but not limited to, — errors, omissions, or inaccuracies.

SPECIAL BONUS!

Want This Bonus Book for FREE?

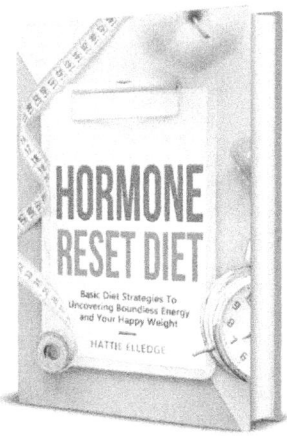

Get **FREE**, unlimited access to it and all of my new books by joining the Fan Base!

Scan me!

CONTENTS

INTRODUCTION

"The food you eat can be either the safest and most powerful form of medicine or the slowest form of poison."
-Ann Wigmore

Let's paint a picture. It's midday and you just finished lunch. Your morning was productive and the rest of the day looms ahead. Whatever you have to accomplish, it's going to take a lot of energy and willpower to finish. So, when you get back to your office, continue your work. Then the crash hits you. A wave of sudden exhaustion rolls over you like a tidal wave, forcing you beneath the water. Your head begins to ache and your brain feels like it's somewhere in the clouds. Suddenly, your tasks seem impossible. All you can think about is lying down somewhere dark. You may pop some ibuprofen and make a cup of coffee in an attempt to shake it off. But it doesn't help and you struggle until you go to bed, hoping tomorrow will bring new energy.

Sound familiar? Everyone has experienced a midday crash at some point in their lives. Most people chalk it up to food but never examine what they ate or how it affects their bodies. They say phrases like, "food makes me sleepy," or

"I ate too much at lunch and just couldn't wake up." They continue on struggling, day after day, never understanding why they feel this way. But the truth is that it's not natural for food to make you tired. It's not normal to crash midday if you had a full night's rest. Our culture has largely accepted exhaustion and lethargy as "common," especially as we age. We are told our bodies and minds begin their descent as we climb over the years. Yes, our metabolism naturally slows the older we get, but it shouldn't look like rapidly increasing health problems.

Maybe you've struggled with a sudden weight change and don't understand where it came from. Perhaps your moods send you into a spiraling depression that takes weeks to recover from, and no medication you try seems to fix the problem. Perhaps the sex drive you once had simply isn't there anymore, and you haven't felt sexy in a long time. There are a million things you could be experiencing: hair loss, infertility, anxiety, depression, fatigue, brain fog, migraines, insomnia, endometriosis... The list is long, but there'll be more on that later. There are a million reasons you could be reading this book. You are not alone. There is hope for a better future.

Because what if there was a way to reclaim your life, body, and health without having to feel the side effects of medication? What if you could lose the weight, and keep it off, without having a procedure or going on a highly restrictive diet? What if you could feel the energy you used to have and reclaim your happiness and life? Well, be assured you absolutely can. But we need to start by understanding just how our hormones work, and what roles they play in our bodies. We also need to understand our food and activities' significance on our bodily chemicals.

There is a difference between being conscious of food and its properties, and diet culture. We are told that fat is bad but lean meat is good. So, you find a diet, stick to it for a few months, and drop a couple of pounds. Maybe you even feel energized again. Then you're off the diet and suddenly, the weight reappears as your energy levels disappear. Why? There are a lot of reasons that we will cover later on. We live in a culture where food is seen as a form of entertainment, not essential fuel for energy. We "diet" because we want a fast and easy solution.

Let me give you another example: you go to the doctor because you have constant migraines, low energy, and you're steadily gaining weight. They tell you that you're "normal," but still prescribe you something to help with the headaches. You fill it, begin taking it, and your headaches aren't as bad. But your energy is still low, and the weight is still there. You're happy to not have headaches, sure, but you wanted this pill to fix all of the problems. Why didn't it work?

Because, while modern medicine is more than necessary, it has entirely replaced the concept of health. We have prescribed medication that covers up symptoms but doesn't heal the actual problem. In other words, we're slapping band-aids over bullet holes and wondering why we're still bleeding.

This isn't about a diet. This is about a lifestyle change. It's about understanding the role our hormones play in our bodies, and the role food plays in our lives. It's about knowing that the chemicals in and on food can affect the chemicals that send messages to the most vital organs in our systems. It's about changing the way you think about food, reclaiming your life, and loving your body.

This book comes from real-life experience in balancing hormones through natural avenues. It stems from a passion to share knowledge and help others live a full, rediscovered life. It comes after navigating through doctor after doctor for each one to say the same thing: "Your levels are in the normal range. Nothing is wrong with you." There is nothing quite as frustrating as not feeling "normal," yet being told you are. Your body tells you when something is wrong, in the same way, your car will turn on that dreaded "check engine" light when it has a problem. If you feel like something is wrong, there is a good chance you're right. This book is full of first-hand experience regarding the chemicals in hormones and food. Here, we take the necessary steps to improve our health. We will also learn what hormones are, their key roles in our bodies, and the science behind balancing them naturally. You will discover the impactful role hormones have on our bodies, how our relationship with food can dramatically alter them, and natural solutions. Let's learn to live our lives and love ourselves again.

MY CHEMICAL MESSENGERS UNDERSTANDING HORMONES

"Medicine is not healthcare-- food is healthcare. Medicine is sickcare. Let's all get this straight for a change." - Anonymous

To understand why diet is so important for our hormones, we need to understand what hormones are and why they are so important in our bodies. Hormones are the "chemical messengers" of our bodies. They are busy, little talkers, affecting all kinds of processes that happen in our bodies. They can alter our growth, development, sexual functions, reproductive systems, and mood. They hold so much power over our bodies, as they are the ones who inform our cells of what is going on and what to produce. Their biggest job is to have a constant, internal conversation with all of our cells and major organs. They are constantly talking to our bodies, telling them what we need and what we don't, so if they are unhappy, your body won't be either.

So, where do these important, microscopic communicators come from? Hormones are produced from endocrine glands, which are found all over your body as well. The pituitary, pineal, thymus, thyroid, adrenals, pancreas, testes, and ovaries are all endocrine glands that produce hormones. So, hormones are produced in all areas of our bodies into our bloodstream, which means they can travel fairly fast and extremely far. The messages they send our bodies are important, because while they are small, there are many, and the messages they relay are powerful.

But what messages should they be sending? According to studies conducted by the Society for Endocrinology, "Hormones have two types of communication in the human body: communication between two endocrine glands and communication between an endocrine gland and a target organ" (Society for Endocrinology, 2021). Endocrine gland to endocrine gland communication is all about changing the level of the hormone being produced. They can lower it or raise it depending on the message the hormone sends.

Endocrine to organ communication directly affects the organ that is targeted. It can raise or lower the levels of hormones in whichever organ it is communicating with.

We're starting to see just how vital a role our hormones have in our health, but we still need to understand their nature and chemical makeup. According to the National Cancer Institute, "Chemical hormones are classified as either proteins or steroids," (Seers, 2021). Most of the hormones that circulate in the human body are proteins or a derivative of a protein. Sex hormones and the hormones produced from the adrenal cortex are steroidal. This means hormones can have various mechanisms depending on their type of chemical makeup.

Let's look at action hormones, for example. The action hormones are the ones that are carried in the bloodstream and have a wide range of movement, but they only influence certain cells. The cells which respond to this hormone do so through a sort of "lock-and-key-mechanism" response. If the hormone matches the specific cell, that cell will have a response. If the hormone and cell don't fit, there is no response. And here's the crazy thing: all cells in our bodies have a receptor site for specific hormones. The receptor site is what is called "target tissue" for the hormone to find. Sometimes, target tissue is found in just a singular gland or organ. Other times, target tissue can be broken up and sent throughout our bodies. This is a huge range of our bodies that hormones can affect.

There are also different ways in which the hormones respond to those receptors. According to the National Cancer Institute, "Protein hormones react with receptors on the surface of the cell, and the sequence of events that results in hormone action is relatively rapid. Steroid hormones typically react with receptor sites inside a cell. This method of action involves synthesis and proteins, so it is relatively slow," (Seers, 2021). In other words, our protein hormones are the changes we can feel or see regularly. Steroid hormones are the ones that cause things like puberty or menopause and develop over time.

Not only do our hormones send messages to our entire system, but they are extremely sensitive, as well. Hormones are powerful because they are highly concentrated. This means that many organs in our bodies have a small limit of the hormone they can receive. See, our bodies work with a constant feedback system. In the same way, products will change depending on user reactions, internally, our organs do the same thing. But instead of being happy with the final product, our bodies stay on a feedback loop. This is a "biological occurrence wherein the output of a system amplifies the system (positive) or inhibits the system (negative)," (Seers, 2021).

Because our hormones are so concentrated, they are often on a negative feedback loop. They are constantly adjusting to stay in the exact amount our body needs. Our hormones are always working for that state of balance, or homeostasis, so we can live and function healthily. Due to their sensitivity and hyperawareness, they can often over or underreact to numerous factors. This can affect our metabolic process and throw homeostasis out. So, although our hormones need to remain in an exact quantity at any given time, it is a difficult thing to maintain.

Okay, so we have a basic understanding of what hormones are, where they come from, and how they function. But what causes those hormones to react and throw our bodies out of homeostasis? What does it look like when that happens? Simply put, "A hormone imbalance occurs when your hormones aren't communicating properly and your body incorrectly produces too much or too little of any hormone," (Parsley Health, 2019). Remember when we said that hormones are constantly communicating with each other? They communicate to achieve homeostasis. They are also communicating when one hormone becomes unbalanced. The unbalanced hormone will send a message to a correlating hormone. In response, that hormone will start producing more or less depending on the messages received. The instability of one hormone can create a snowball effect in your system, wreaking havoc on your body.

We've all heard how stress is a major factor in hormone imbalance, but it can cause major changes to our hormones. Stress correlates with our thyroid, which is where cortisol is produced. When our body feels stressed, it enters "flight or fight" mode, which increases our cortisol production. The cortisol hormone has a direct influence on the immune system, nervous system, pancreas, liver, and fat tissues. Constant exposure to high cortisol levels can lead to chronic fatigue, irritability, mood swings, and weight gain.

But, as previously stated, everyone knows stress affects your hormones. Consider the impact chronic inflammation can have on those chemical messengers. Chronic inflammation can mess with numerous systems in your body. It can influence your testosterone, insulin production, and cortisol. High cortisol can mess with female hormone imbalance, in particular, being one of the leading causes of PCOS. It can also decrease the production of ovarian hormones. This can heavily have negative effects on your menstrual cycle, such as extreme PMS and painful cycles. Inflammation is directly linked to gut health, as you will see with so many other root causes.

Your blood sugar levels are another factor that can correlate to hormone imbalance. Many people suffer from low blood sugar daily, and never even realize it. When your blood sugar plummets, it produces adrenaline. (Parsley Health, 2019). This adrenaline enters your bloodstream and triggers your stress hormone, cortisol. Then, both adrenaline and cortisol relay a message to your pituitary gland located in your brain, and this triggers your "fight or flight" mode. In response, your brain lowers your sex hormone production to conserve energy for more vital bodily functions. (Parsley Health, 2019). If you consume a lot of processed foods with no true nutritional value, your blood sugar levels could be getting thrown off.

Believe it or not, the environment is also a leading cause of hormone imbalance. In today's day and age, innovation is the key to success. We are surrounded by new products and new technology. And just when you think you've caught up, someone somewhere creates a newer version. While innovation is great, and science is amazing, have you ever thought about the chemical components of the products you're using? Or the chemicals sprayed on the vegetables you're eating? Or the additives in food, which give them longer shelf time? Pesticides, additives, herbicides, and synthetic materials containing xenoestrogens, can infiltrate your endocrine system (Talida, 2021). Xenoestrogens act like estrogen in the body, sending a message to estrogen to halt production. This can tax your liver function and iron levels, causing weight gain and major mood swings.

Speaking of iron levels, another root cause for hormonal imbalance lies in our nutrients. Did you know that your gut contains more neurotransmitters than your brain? (Parsley Health, 2019). Our stomachs are more than vital to every component of our health. Our gut receives information, in the same way, our brain receives information, but it receives more. Our intestines are made to process our food by separating the need from the waste and moving both to the proper areas in our bodies. The gut is lined with microbiomes, which are small microorganisms that help us process everything which enters our bacterial system (Parsley health, 2019). It receives messages from our food, environment, and thought process, and uses that information to make decisions on the hormones the body needs more or less of.

So, what if the food you eat doesn't contain any nutrients your body needs? Your body can get confused. Even though you're eating, if it doesn't contain what your gut and overall system needs, it could begin to store it, because it thinks you are starving. The toxicity from nutrient deficiency can also build up over time. Because here's the deal: "Nutrients form the building blocks of our hormones. We cannot have adequate hormone production without the nutrients to create them," (Parsley Health, 2019). In other words, if we are starved of proper nutrients, our hormones begin to starve as well. They will stop producing, and when one hormone stops producing, all the other hormones will respond. This creates toxicity in our bodies or a hormonal imbalance.

If you're sitting here thinking, well great, everything can cause a hormonal imbalance, don't worry. There are ways to naturally achieve hormonal balance and regain your energy and health. I will warn you: it takes hard work, dedication, and an honest review of your lifestyle. Because what you put into your body, is one-hundred percent, what you will get out of your body. In the same way that sending the right communication to a partner is vital to a healthy relationship, sending the right communication to your body is vital to your health. All of this begins in your mind. Your brain controls everything, and whether or not you believe this is possible - you're right. Let's look at the mindset changes which need to occur in order to achieve hormonal balance and feel alive again.

This is not about controlling every single thing you eat. This is about being conscious of what you're putting into your body. It's about your relationship with food and how you view it. Food is fuel. It is what our "engines" run on, and how we survive day-to-day. It is nothing else. And you deserve a clean, well-oiled engine that doesn't threaten to break down on you every hundred miles. You deserve to have the energy, body, and mind which keeps you active and happy every day. Oftentimes, our relationship with food is a direct reflection of our relationship with ourselves. If you control every morsel of everything you eat, you probably feel like you have to control every aspect of your life in order to be happy. Your body will respond to this. If you think you are undeserving of good things, and eat bad food all of the time to feel better, your body will respond to this. The truth is, it's easy to use food as a defense mechanism in any situation. But shifting this mindset, whatever your case, can and will change your life.

This isn't to say you can't enjoy food. In fact, it's quite the opposite. Food doesn't have to taste disgusting in order for it to be healthy. Being conscious of what you're eating, knowing you are bettering yourself, and eating the way your body needs, is often the most enjoyable thing to do. But how do you know what your body needs? What are the right foods to help your body achieve homeostasis?

The food your body needs in order to get the correct nutrients can vary slightly from person to person, but overall, there are some great ways to get started eating the right "fuel food." First, carbs are not bad, they simply should be balanced. Our bodies turn macronutrients (carbs, fats, and proteins) into energy! Now, finding the right carbs, fats, and proteins is different, but we'll get into that in a minute. Fermented foods and foods containing high fiber are also extremely important for balancing hormones.

Another mindset change we need to have regarding diet is the way we look at fat. In the 1950s, research emerged linking saturated fat and cholesterol with heart disease (Happy Hormones, 2020). After this, the low-fat industry began and has been booming ever since. This research has now been invalidated, and more people are realizing just how important healthy fats are to achieve a balanced system. Yes, there are plenty of unhealthy, fat products out there, but this is because they are typically trans fats, paired with enriched wheat flour and hydrogenated oil. Your body cannot break down any of these ingredients, let alone turn them into nutrients. But healthy fats are so important for your hormones and your body.

When the "Low Fat Fad" hit the market, a lot of things happened to our food that impacted our health. First, taking fat out of the food also took the nutrients along with it, including fat-soluble vitamins like A, D, E, and K. Second, the taste of fat needed to be replaced, so oftentimes, processed sugars or artificial flavoring (chemicals) were used. Third, going low-fat means unintentionally going high-carb, which spikes your blood sugar and can throw your hormones out of balance. This can lead to excess insulin, over-eating because your body is starved of the correct nutrients, which then will lead to fat-storing. (Happy Hormones, 2020).

To this day, many people are not fully aware of the benefits of healthy fat. But your brain is made up of sixty percent fat, which contains neurotransmitters and signals your hormone pathways. If you are starved of such nutrients, your brain will not have the correct messages to send to your hormones. Additionally, every cell you have requires fat so the membranes can function correctly. One of these functions includes helping hormones target and enter the correct cells. Fat also helps your body absorb those fat-soluble vitamins that are so vital for your hormones to transmit correct messages. Lastly, healthy fats can greatly improve your cholesterol, which is a major factor in your steroid hormones. It is also important for your body to be able to produce vitamin D! (Happy Hormones, 2020).

Healthy fats include salmon, avocado, nuts and seeds, grass-fed meat, coconut oil, olive oil, and even butter (when not paired with unhealthy foods). Eating some of these products on a daily basis can greatly improve your energy, and also begin to help regulate your hormones. High-fiber foods can also be beneficial. Fruits and legumes can help your body further break down nutrients, supporting your hormone health. Fermented foods naturally contain probiotics that boost hormone regularity.

Another great start to balancing hormones naturally, is to find an exercise routine that works for you. Our bodies are incredible. It is one system with many parts that all collaborate to carry out a goal. Everything inside of us is connected. According to Dr. Amy Lee, "The amount of movement and physical activity we do on a daily basis makes a huge impact on the hormonal responses of the body," (Lawrenson, 2021). Exercise can increase the hormones which keep you lean and strong like, testosterone, HGH, and progesterone.

Dr. Lee gives a great example of this when she tells us, "When we contract our muscle fibers, the movement and fiber activation communicate with the fat cells and adipose tissues by hormonal signaling. Our heart rate and the activation of our nervous system also cause our brain to release various hormones which ultimately control how our peripheral organs respond," (Lawrenson, 2021). So, exercise is extremely important for our lifestyle if we want to balance our hormones naturally. It's important to note that working out too much is not good for your hormones, either. Your body is constantly communicating with you. Listen to when it tells you to rest, and when it tells you to push harder. Our systems know what we need and will usually let us know when we need to rest.

Sleep, caffeine intake, and water intake are huge factors in balancing hormones. Lack of sleep can affect your cortisol levels in the same way stress does. Cortisol is often thought of as a "negative hormone" but like all hormones in our body, it is necessary during some periods. However, we want to control our cortisol levels to release only when we really need them - in high-stress situations (Lawrenson, 2021). Caffeine also has the same effect as stress and sleep. Getting too much caffeine daily can increase cortisol levels, as well. Limiting caffeine to one to two servings per day can help in getting your hormones back to normal. Also, increasing your water to sixty-four ounces a day can help balance and flush your system of any toxins messing with your hormones (Chapel Hill Gynecology, 2019).

The bottom line is that there are numerous ways to balance your hormones naturally. It's not unattainable to get your health back, without getting on a prescription! While we have a brief overview of some various ways to get back to your natural hormone balance, we will take a more in-depth dive later on. For now, just know that your endocrine system is complex, vast, and very sensitive. What you put in your body matters, and the way you treat yourself matters, too. But this is just the beginning of amazing discoveries of what your body is capable of when fueled!

Chapter Summary

- Hormones are the chemical messengers of our bodies.
- Hormones can get stuck on a negative feedback loop because they are always fighting for homeostasis.
- Everything in our body is connected and if the messages it's receiving are incorrect, it can cause a wide variety of reactions.

In the next chapter, you will learn….
- How and why hormones are so sensitive.
- What triggers a hormonal imbalance.
- How to deal with your hormones when they are triggered.

WHY SO TRIGGERED?
HORMONAL TRIGGERS AND
WHAT TO DO ABOUT THEM

"A fresh start isn't a new place, it's a new mindset." -
Anonymous

Now we know what hormones are, how the endocrine
system works, some root causes for hormonal imbalances,
and have a good overview of the natural remedies that work.
But we need to dive deeper. Let's look at what a hormonal
imbalance really is, and the signs you might have. According
to Healthline, "Hormonal imbalances stem from your body
making too much or too little of a hormone or series of
hormones," (Healthline, 2020). And we know that even the
slightest change can have drastic effects all over the human
body. And while hormones do change with age, if your

endocrine glands are getting the wrong signals, then your entire body will let you know.

There are also different types of hormonal imbalances which have to do with the different hormones that could be receiving the wrong signal. The first we are going to look at is a cortisol imbalance. To review, cortisol is the "flight or fight" hormone produced in the adrenal glands. Cortisol regulates blood sugar, metabolism, inflammation, and memory formation. But, remember, cortisol is our stress hormone, so if this hormone is released for a long period of time, it can temporarily shut down your digestion and reproduction system (Medical Group, 2021).

There are many symptoms of a cortisol imbalance, varying whether or not high cortisol or low cortisol. If your adrenal gland is pumping too much cortisol into your system, you could develop a red and round face, weight gain, extreme thirst, weak muscles, irregular menstruation, low sex drive, and high blood sugar. On the other hand, low cortisol can elicit symptoms such as rapid weight loss, fatigue, muscle weakness, mood swings, and dizziness (Medical Group, 2021).

Estrogen is another hormonal imbalance that could be affecting your health. Now, estrogen is predominately associated with women, as it is their main sex hormone, but men also secrete estrogen, just in smaller doses. An estrogen imbalance is more likely to occur in women, however, it can occur in men, as well. In women, estrogen is responsible for puberty, and a regular menstrual cycle. It also supports their bones and heart health during pregnancy. But in both men and women, estrogen balances bone health and cholesterol (Medical Group, 2021).

High estrogen can cause a number of problems such as weight gain, tender breasts, or lumps in your breasts, depression, and anxiety, and weight gain. Low estrogen "symptoms" in women is often just the beginning of menopause. But in others, including men, things like hot flashes, dry and itchy skin, mood swings, and low libido (Medical Group, 2021).

Another hormonal imbalance we are going to look at is insulin imbalance. Insulin is made in your pancreas. Insulin directly affects your liver, fat, and muscles. It helps these things break down nutrients such as fat, protein, and sugar. This is how your metabolic process stays in check and keeps you energized and healthy. So, what does an insulin imbalance look like? In low insulin, Type One and Two diabetes are often the results. People with diabetes are more likely to experience high insulin effects if they accidentally inject too much (Medical Group, 2021).

Next, we will look at a testosterone hormonal imbalance. While testosterone is the male sex hormone, women have testosterone too, only in smaller amounts. Like estrogen in women, testosterone is the cause of puberty in men. However, in women, testosterone is important for healthy, strong bones and their reproductive tissue. There are many concerning symptoms of both high and low testosterone in both men and women (Medical group, 2021).

High testosterone in men can make them exhibit aggressive behavior, and cause or worsen sleep apnea. They will often show signs of an increase in their muscular tissue. It also puts them at risk to become infertile when they are younger. Low testosterone can greatly affect men but women, as well. In men, it also increases the chances of infertility because it can lower their sperm count. It can also cause symptoms such as irritable mood, low sex drive, and trouble keeping erections. In women, the lowering of the testosterone hormone can cause issues like extreme fatigue, low sex drive, weight gain, and weakened muscles (Medical Group, 2021).

The final hormone imbalance we are going to look at is a progesterone imbalance. Progesterone is another hormone mostly linked to females, but men also have it. It helps to balance fertility in both males and females and is extremely vital for women during the first trimester of pregnancy. For men, it is important because it helps regulate their estrogen levels (Medical Group, 2021).

High progesterone can cause an array of problems in men. If progesterone rises, estrogen will react, rising to match the level of the progesterone. This can lead to symptoms like fatigue and depression. It can also put men at risk to develop heart problems. In women, it causes instability in weight, anxiety, low sex drive, and bloating. On the other hand, low testosterone in men can have an effect on their bone density. Other symptoms may include, early hair loss, weight gain, and fatigue. In women, low progesterone is highly dangerous during early pregnancies. In fact, low levels of progesterone have been linked to miscarriages, as well as painful pregnancies. Other symptoms include an irregular menstrual cycle, and low sex drive (Medical Group, 2021).

Now that we have gone over a lot of the science behind our hormones and what certain imbalances can cause, let's look at some of the major myths we hear surrounding our hormones. The truth is, if your hormones are balanced in a way that is right for you, many of the common things we hear in regards to hormones simply aren't true. There are over two hundred hormones in your body, and everyone's nutritional needs for those hormones are unique. According to the Institute for Integrative Nutrition, "There is not a one-size-fits-all diet. Each person is a unique individual with highly individualized requirements. This is known as bio-individuality," (Rosenthal, 2019). By dissecting the myths, we can reflect on our own lifestyles and habits in order to begin to understand our bio-individuality.

The first myth we are going to debunk involves the notorious soy. It's commonly believed that soy should be avoided for hormonal health, especially by women. Various studies conducted in the late nineties liked soy to lower cholesterol and overall heart health. However, many food companies monopolized this and began adding "heart-healthy" to their soy products. Today, more studies focus on the hormonal impacts of consuming soy. But why is soy so commonly linked to bad hormones? Because soy contains a chemical found in plants called phytoestrogen. Soy's specific type of phytoestrogen is called an isoflavone (Integrative Nutrition, 2021).

These isoflavones are concentrated versions of phytoestrogens. This means they are structurally similar to estrogen and can mimic hormones, but they are not as strong as the actual hormone. While this isn't always a bad thing - it can promote bone strength and small amounts can prevent breast cancer - its behavior is complicated enough to be problematic. Because these isoflavones can mimic hormones, sometimes they can take over actual estrogen. According to The Institute for Integrative Nutrition, "They can bind to those estrogen, hormone receptors and block their activation, which can hinder processes that require estrogen," (Integrative Nutrition, 2021).

However, this does not mean soy is bad for overall hormonal health. The effects of soy on estrogen production depend upon an individual person's own estrogen production and chemicals. Soy is a bio-individual product, and there are many recent studies that have linked small, daily, soy consumption to a lower risk for breast cancer. If you maintain a balanced, health-conscious diet, it is more likely that consuming small amounts of soy won't hinder your hormone health (Integrative Nutrition, 2021).

Another huge myth surrounding hormone imbalance is that men don't need to worry about it. Hormones are so often associated with women alone, but hormones play a major role in men's health as well. We know that men have more of the sex hormone, testosterone, than women. But just how important is this hormone? For men, testosterone is key for their muscle mass, sex drive, bone health, and sperm production. An imbalance in this hormone can cause major issues for men later on. Their hormonal changes might not be as abrupt as women's, but this does not mean it's not something they should watch for or think about (Integrative Nutrition, 2021).

The next myth we are going to address is one of the

most widely believed ones in our world today. It's the belief that the only way to treat hormonal imbalances is through medication because we have no control over our hormones. Of course, there are certain medical conditions and different situations which do require a type of hormone therapy. But there are natural routes most people can take in order to get back in control of their hormones.

Like we said before, what you put into your body, is what you get out of it. But to take that even further, "Food has the power to heal- or harm - our bodies," (Rosenthal, 2019). So, if food has the power to heal or harm our bodies, then it can absolutely heal or harm our hormones. If we think about hormones like leptin, ghrelin, and insulin, we see that they correlate to the sugars and carbs we consume on a daily basis, because these hormones are responsible for the regulation of blood sugars, as well as signaling our brain when we're hungry.

Let's take a look at the fast-food industry. Beginning in 1948, with the staple McDonald's, it has now grown into a $200 billion dollar annual revenue industry. It has altered our countries' eating habits and chemically changed food production. (Food is Power, 2021). Fast food is filled with sodium, chemically processed sugars, and high-saturated fats and oils. It has led to an unspoken epidemic in our world: obesity. If we are to weigh the opposite of fast food, true sustenance that nurtures our bodies, the chemical composition is vastly different from that of fast food.

If a person's diet is made up of fast food, or processed sugars, and saturated fat, these chemicals are going to directly affect our own chemicals. Let's look at our "hunger hormones," for example. The hormone ghrelin is responsible for sending messages to our brain to alert it of hunger. On the opposite side of ghrelin is the hormone, leptin. Leptin is responsible for telling our brain when we are full, or satisfied. Studies found that overweight individuals developed leptin resistance, which caused the leptin hormone to elevate its levels. This confuses the messages the brain receives from the hormone and overeating occurs as a result. Both of these hunger hormones require a balanced diet in order for them to perform properly. Eating sugary and inflammatory foods can throw these hormones off balance easily (Medical Group, 2021).

Another example lies in the insulin hormone. Processed sugar is influential on our insulin production and response. If an individual's diet is one of high, processed sugar, our body will react by attempting to flush the sugar out of the blood cells. But the sugar has already saturated these cells, so instead of being processed through our liver, our liver stores it as fat, even though our liver's main function is to help detoxify our body (Medical Group, 2021). Think of your liver like a glass of water, but once the glass of water that empties once it becomes full. But when your body's hormones become confused, impure water can be sent to this water glass. The glass of water doesn't recognize it as normal water, so instead of dumping it, it stores the toxin. If this happens enough times, that glass of water can become full of impure water. Now, it doesn't have room for the good water, because it doesn't know what to do with the bad. This can cause a negative reaction throughout your entire body.

The bottom line is that we can absolutely control our hormones. Not in every case, but in many cases, changing our lifestyle and eating habits can have a positive impact on the body's functions and hormones. Your hormones need to be nurtured correctly in order to function properly.

Most women believe menopause won't become an issue until they are over fifty, however, this is not always the case. Menopause can happen much later than your early fifties, or much earlier. There is also a transition called the premenopausal stage, which a woman goes through before menopause can happen. These symptoms can last up to four years before menopause kicks in! Most believe they have to have hormone therapy medications in order to ease the symptoms of menopause. However, eating foods that are anti-inflammatory and finding more natural supplements can be extremely beneficial to a woman going through menopause. The truth is that everyone's experience is not going to be the same, so understanding our bodies and hormones can help a woman navigate this stage in her life and continue to feel healthy and energetic (Integrative Nutrition, 2021).

Another myth that is important to debunk is the belief in adrenal fatigue. It's a common belief in our society that adrenal fatigue or chronic fatigue, means a person is overworked or just "burned out." However, this is not the case. Adrenal fatigue occurs when our adrenal glands become overworked and stop functioning efficiently. See, our adrenals are responsible for secreting hormones that regulate your stress reactions, metabolism, and blood pressure levels. When your adrenals are taxed, you can have symptoms like, chronic fatigue, craving salty food, feeling unmotivated, and brain fog. The biggest problem with "adrenal fatigue" is that it is not easily diagnosed when someone is experiencing these symptoms. Oftentimes, people will be told that they are just "stressed and overworked" when they are really experiencing adrenal fatigue. The good news is that by changing your diet and finding supplements that work for you, adrenal fatigue can be easily fixed (Integrative Nutrition, 2021).

Now, let's look at the myths surrounding postpartum depression. Most women who go through this believe it's their fault, or it will go away on its own. It's vital to note that experiencing postpartum depression is extremely common, and never the woman's fault. One in thirteen women will experience PPD after having a child! The more sensitive one's hormones are, the more at risk a person is to have PPD. This does not mean there is something wrong with you. It is a chemical imbalance your body is having after all of the hormones you had from the baby (Peternell, 2020).

Postpartum depression will not go away on its own, in most cases. However, there are lifestyle changes and help one can get in order to get back to their normal hormones. It's recommended that a woman suffering from PPD find cognitive behavior therapy because it has been proven to positively affect the symptoms of PPD. Foods with omega-3 fatty acids can also help with PPD, as well as acupuncture and massage therapy (Peternell, 2020). PPD is not a hopeless cause and not something you should suffer in silence from. There are plenty of ways to remedy the hormonal imbalance after having a baby.

The final myth we are going to address is for the girls, and it's the lie of tolerating PMS. Premenstrual Syndrome, or PMS, is largely accepted as normal, but the symptoms are vast and the severity can be brutal. You do not have to accept this as normal! Numerous studies have proven that vitamin B6, calcium, vitamin E, and magnesium can alleviate PMS symptoms. You can achieve this through either diet or supplementation, but both are highly recommended. Vitamin B has proven to help with that awful moodiness that PMS can bring on. Foods like fish, chicken, and starches contain high concentrations of Vitamin B. Calcium can help during the luteal phase of your cycle as well, proven to reduce food cravings and anxiety. Vitamin E is beneficial to the skin and muscles and can reduce breast tenderness. Magnesium relaxes the muscles helping with headaches and cramps (Integrative Nutrition, 2021). There is no reason you have to accept PMS as a normal occurrence every month. There are natural ways, through supplements and diet, to help you live without having to deal with horrible PMS.

Although we have had a brief overview of what some signs of a hormonal imbalance might look like, we need to take a deeper dive into all the signs and symptoms one can experience. Because each gender has different amounts of certain hormones, we need to separate the signs in both. Let's start with men.

Because men only have high levels of one sex hormone, as opposed to women, the effects of a hormonal imbalance in men are often more gradual than in women (Center for

Healing, 2021). However, this does not mean that their symptoms are any less. First, there is research linked to lack of sleep and type two diabetes in men. As men's natural testosterone decreases as they age, their cortisol levels respond to this change by decreasing their levels, as well. The research found that testosterone and cortisol can reduce the negative effects caused by lack of sleep, therefore, decreasing the risk of developing type two diabetes. That aside, a general list of signs men can have if they have a hormonal imbalance are as follows: weight loss or gain, dry skin, extreme thirst, headaches, fatigue, mood swings, depression, profuse sweating, anxiety, blood pressure changes, and blood sugar changes (Center for Healing, 2021).

Women often have to be more aware of their hormones, as hormones are what control their menstrual cycles and pregnancy. However, a hormonal imbalance still can be easily missed, because women's hormones fluctuate on a monthly basis, and oftentimes they can think they are just experiencing an "off month," when in reality it could be the beginning of a hormonal imbalance. It is very important to catch these imbalances, as even the slightest hormonal imbalance can lead to serious problems like ovarian cancer or early menopause. Some signs of a hormonal imbalance in women are as follows: irregular or missed periods, low sex drive, infertility, sudden or unexplained weight gain, mood swings, bloating, and insomnia (Center for Healing, 2021).

Identifying the different types of hormonal imbalances helps us be able to recognize the ones we could be dealing with, and how to deal with them. We now understand that controlling is possible, and nutrition and diet is the key to success. Understanding the myths of hormone imbalance is important, because it opens our eyes to the truth behind hormones and how varied an individual's experience can be. Being aware of the signs and symptoms of hormonal imbalance helps keep us in tune with our bodies, so we can identify when we feel "off." Now, instead of brushing it away as "being overworked," we can take action against hormonal imbalances so they don't get worse. These are all important factors if we are going to try to regulate our hormones naturally!

Chapter Summary

+ Different hormones control different functions in our body.
+ Different hormones can cause different types of imbalances.
+ It's important to know and identify the different myths surrounding hormonal imbalance.
+ It is essential to understand what type of hormone imbalance you have in order to know how to handle it.

In the next chapter, you will learn….
+ How age plays a role in hormonal imbalance.
+ The variations of imbalance can come with each age group and gender.
+ How to handle the hormone issues that come with the aging process.

THE AGE OF IT ALL
UNDERSTANDING HOW AGE
AFFECTS HORMONES

"Age is not lost youth but a new stage of opportunity and growth." -Betty Friedan

Now that we know the different types of hormonal imbalances, the myths behind hormones, and the signs and symptoms of experiencing one, we need to take a look at different factors that can play a role. Gender and age are two huge key points in hormonal imbalances. We need to understand how hormonal imbalances act in both genders, as well as how age can drastically affect their symptoms and signs. Because hormonal imbalances can affect everyone from adolescence to senior years, we will look at the types of hormonal imbalances all ages and genders can experience!

Let's begin with hormone imbalances in adult males. We know that most men tend to accept variations in their bodies as the aging process and sweep the symptoms under the rug. However, as adult males age, these changes are typically linked to hormonal imbalances. According to Dr. Jag Desai, with the Core Medical and Wellness Center, "Male growth hormones tend to steadily decrease after age twenty, and by age forty, most men retain only half of their original growth hormones, and by eighty, they typically only retain 5%," (Desai, 2019). So, while we can clearly see that age is a major factor, there are many other contributing factors to hormonal imbalances in adult males. Things like activity level, poor diet and nutrition, medications, prolonged exposure to stress, injuries, and genetics, should all be taken into account when one is suffering from a hormonal imbalance. Because, aging doesn't have to mean losing your energy, sleep, and proper body functions.

What are some of the common types of hormonal imbalances in adult males? We know that testosterone is the main male hormone, however, there is also cortisol, insulin, and thyroid hormones. An imbalance with any of these four hormones can cause the following four main hormonal imbalances in adult males. Andropause, or 'male menopause,' is caused by testosterone levels dropping too low. Adrenal fatigue can occur when a man is exposed to stress for a long period of time. This can cause his cortisol levels to drop, resulting in overworked adrenal glands. Hypothyroidism is caused by an underactive thyroid gland, which can cause severe joint pain in adult males. Hyperthyroidism is caused by an overactive one, which can often result in major issues later on, such as cancer (Medanta, 2019).

There are many different ways a hormonal imbalance can affect a man's health. In some cases, he can develop gynecomastia or breast enlargement. This is oftentimes chalked up to a bad diet and poor lifestyle. However, a higher level of estrogen than testosterone is the culprit behind this. Low sex drive is another symptom men experiencing a hormonal imbalance can face. If a man's testosterone has dropped, sometimes his sex drive will as well. Erectile dysfunction can be a sign of a testosterone imbalance in a man, but it's often accompanied by other, underlying issues. However, chronic stress can imbalance the cortisol level, resulting in erectile dysfunction (BodyLogic, 2021).

Now, let's look at hormonal imbalances in adult females. There are many hormonal imbalances that occur in adult females that are a natural part of a women's menstrual cycle, pregnancy or menopause, later on in life. However, there are many causes and issues adult females can face with unnatural hormonal issues. And just like men, women can overlook these issues thinking that they are a part of their natural cycle each month (Brennan, 2020).

Adult females can experience issues with their thyroid. Either an overactive or underactive thyroid can cause major problems for women. It could be due to certain medication or an underlying autoimmune disorder. Women can also experience prolonged exposure to stress, which can cause their bodies to produce too much cortisol, for an extended period of time. Eating disorders can also take a toll on the hormone levels in an adult females' body. Nutrition is key is estrogen and progesterone production, and when the body does not receive enough nutrition, estrogen, and progesterone can become dangerously low (Brennan, 2020).

Some common hormone problems adult females face can often majorly interfere with their everyday lives. Irregular or unusually heavy periods can stem from an overproduction of male hormones. This can sometimes lead to Polycystic Ovary Syndrome. If a woman is experiencing a decrease in sex drive or vaginal dryness, low estrogen is the most likely culprit. Thyroid hormones are vital for balancing a woman's body weight, and an imbalance of the thyroid can cause sudden weight gain. For a female adult, progesterone is directly correlated with relaxation and sleep.

A drop in progesterone could cause insomnia, and an increase in progesterone could cause chronic fatigue. Chronic bloating is another major issue that is most likely linked to a hormone imbalance. The cells in a woman's digestive tracts have hormone receptors for estrogen and progesterone. If either one of these hormones becomes unbalanced, bloating, constipation and diarrhea can become a common occurrence. And then we have mood swings, the ever-problematic frustration a woman can face on a monthly basis. While it is normal to experience mood swings during the menstrual cycle or menopause, constant, mood swings can be frustrating and are not normal. This could be due to an underlying thyroid imbalance, and can be fixed (Brennan, 2020).

The next group we are going to examine is adolescent males. While puberty is a part of life and will cause a surge in necessary hormones needed for development, adolescent males can certainly experience unnatural hormonal imbalances. Hormonal imbalances that can alter the release of a needed developmental hormone can cause a hormonal imbalance in adolescent males. This can influence their development, mental health, metabolism, and growth. It is important to catch these hormonal imbalances because they are in some of their most vulnerable and critical years (University Hospitals, 2021).

One of the most common issues adolescent males can face is gynecomastia. This condition occurs when adolescent males develop enlarged breasts. It stems from a deficiency in testosterone during puberty or a rise in estrogen. The good news is that this condition typically corrects itself in two years, however, there are many ways to correct this problem. Another potential hormonal imbalance could be a delay in puberty. If an adolescent male has not developed testicles by age fourteen, it is considered to be a delay. This can mean his testosterone levels are naturally lower and could result in hormone problems later on (University Hospitals, 2021).

One of the most important factors a hormonal imbalance can affect a teenage boy is a mental health. During the early stages of puberty, the hypothalamus creates and secretes gonadotropin. This is the vital hormone that initiates all production for growth, sex, and adrenal hormones. When the levels of each of these hormones increase, it is perfectly normal for an adolescent male to become moody. However, it's important to note that an imbalance in any one of these growth hormones puts a teenage boy at risk for mental health problems. When paired with major stress, a hormonal imbalance can increase the stress hormone receptors, while lowering the relaxation hormone receptors. This can cause an adolescent male to develop a long-term, anxiety disorder (Stonewater, 2021).

Because testosterone is developing at such a rapid pace during a boy's adolescent years, an imbalance can also cause irritability, which can be one of the first signs of poor mental health. Major fluctuations between testosterone and estrogen can result in a teenage boy experiencing confusion, a low sense of self-worth, brain fog, social withdrawal, and waves of excitement. Chronic stress, poor diet and nutrition, and environmental factors are leading causes for hormonal imbalance in adolescent males. There is always an answer for hormonal imbalance, and these causes can be remedied. Maintaining a balanced diet is extremely important for adolescent males in both growth and hormones. Maintaining an active lifestyle can be a good outlet for excess testosterone and help to balance mood. It's important to make sure your teenager is visiting the doctor regularly, to make sure his hormones and health are on the right track for a healthy life (Stonewater, 2021).

Puberty is a difficult time for adolescent females, and an unknown hormonal imbalance can make it much harder. Dealing with their changing bodies and developing hormones often will cause a teenage girl to become moody and secretive, which is normal. However, if more is at play, it can be hard to catch a hormonal imbalance, since the topic is already hard for them to talk about. So how can you tell when a teenage girl is suffering from more than just moodiness? Oftentimes, symptoms of a hormonal imbalance can be visible. A sudden weight gain or delay in puberty are common signs of a hormonal imbalance. If a teenage girl is suddenly experiencing extreme fatigue or developing facial hair, there is most likely a hormonal imbalance at play. Symptoms you might not be able to recognize, like heavy menstrual bleeding or depression and anxiety, also stem from a hormonal imbalance. Many teenage girls do not understand what changes they are going through, and will not recognize the signs of a hormonal imbalance (Coyle Institute, 2021).

Adolescent females have a lot of hormones shifting and changing when they go through puberty. However, the main hormones which are the most likely culprits of hormonal imbalance are progesterone, estrogen, cortisol, thyroid, and testosterone. Progesterone is found in the ovaries and will increase production during ovulation. If an adolescent female's progesterone production drops, she could suffer from irregular periods, increased anxiety, and migraines. If her progesterone gets too high, this can cause estrogen to become the dominant hormone instead of balanced. An estrogen imbalance can cause major issues for a teenage girl. If estrogen becomes dominant, it will increase production. Too much estrogen can cause horrible PMS, extreme moodiness, weight gain, and tender breasts. On the other hand, not enough estrogen can cause chronic UTIs, body aches, fatigue, hot flashes, and brain fog (Coyle Institute, 2021).

Now, we know cortisol is a vital hormone to everyone, but in the formative years of a female, the balance of this hormone is extremely important. In a teenage girl, too much cortisol can cause Cushing's Disease, and extreme anxiety and depression. But low cortisol levels could cause Addison's disease, which is what occurs when the adrenal glands do not produce enough hormones, leading to fatigue, dizziness, and weight loss. And any fluctuation in the thyroid can become a prominent issue for teenage girls. Hyperthyroidism, when too much thyroid hormone is secreted, heart palpitations, drastic weight loss, fatigue, and anxiety can occur. Hypothyroidism, when not enough thyroid hormone is present, weight gain, dry skin, irregular periods, and depression can occur. Teenage girls also develop testosterone in small amounts during puberty. Too much testosterone is most likely the underlying issue behind PCOS (Coyle Institution, 2021).

Like adolescent males, hormone imbalances can also take a toll on a teenage girl's mental health. For a girl, estrogen levels are directly in charge of serotonin, which is a neurotransmitter in the brain. If estrogen is too low, then in response, serotonin levels will drop, leading to depression. If estrogen is too high, this could lead to mood instability and irritability (Stonewater, 2021). For adolescent females, and endocrine gland malfunction could be the cause behind many of these hormonal imbalances. Because the endocrine impacts our hormone production, puberty can cause hormones to go awry, influencing the way our endocrine gland functions. Just like in teenage boys, making sure an adolescent girl has a balanced diet with lots of nutrition is vital to her hormonal health. Staying active will also help balance her hormones and her mental state. A teenage girl should also see a doctor regularly to discuss any issues with her menstrual cycle, body, or health. Hormonal health is one of the most important in development, and keeping track of it is always the safest way to go (Coyle Institution, 2021).

The last groups we will be taking a look at are senior men and women. People over the age of fifty are much more likely to experience hormonal imbalances, but why? According to John E. Morley, M.B., "Levels of most hormones decrease with age, but some hormones remain at the same levels typical of those in younger adults, and some even increase," (Morley, 2019). So, even if some remain the same, and some increase, your endocrine system will still be impacted by aging, because as you age, your hormone receptors become less sensitive (Morley, 2019).

Hormone levels most likely to decrease are the growth hormone, melatonin, testosterone, and estrogen. Then we have the hormones most likely to stay the same. These are insulin, thyroid hormones, and cortisol. The hormones most likely to increase are follicle-stimulating hormones, parathyroid hormone, and norepinephrine (Morley, 2019). But what does all of this mean? How does this affect a person's body? There are many ways the decrease of some hormones and the increase of others can play out, but let's go over the most obvious ones.

We've all heard of menopause, but what is it really? Women, around the age of fifty, experience a decrease in estrogen and progesterone. Their ovaries stop making as much, resulting in the pituitary gland overcompensating by making more follicle-stimulating hormones (Rush, 2021). While this is a normal part of the aging process, it is still a hormonal imbalance that can create a list of unwanted symptoms. Most women experience insomnia, decreased libido, mood swings and depression, vaginal dryness leading to painful intercourse, hot flashes, and even osteoporosis (Rush, 2021).

Just because this is a reality every woman will have to face does not mean she must learn to live with the symptoms. Although a study in the early 2000's revealed issues with the prescribed, long-term use of an estrogen, progesterone combination that was used to help manage the symptoms of menopause, does not mean that there is no help. Another recent study revealed that taking these hormones, in small doses, for short periods of time is safe. However, there are natural remedies to help manage menopause. A balanced diet, regular physical activity, and stress management can help alleviate symptoms. Black cohosh, a natural herb, can be used to help manage sleep disturbances and hot flashes. Magnesium can also be helpful in mood stability and relaxation. Almost seventy-five percent of women are deficient in magnesium, and it also begins to decrease with age. Supplementing this with a natural vitamin can be extremely beneficial to women going through menopause. Techniques such as controlled breathing and acupuncture can be extremely beneficial in mood stability, sleeping patterns, and hot flashes. Eating foods high in Omega 3, like fish with high-fat content, can delay the onset of menopause (Boss, 2018).

Senior men can experience andropause, however, not all men go through this. While andropause is sometimes referred to as "male menopause," that's not really the case. All women will go through menopause at some point in their life. Only twenty percent of men over the age of sixty, and thirty to fifty percent of men over the age of eighty will go through andropause. Andropause is when the body experiences a significant drop in the production of testosterone. It can significantly alter a man's well-being and day-to-day life (Rush, 2021).

Andropause can cause a man to develop a low sex drive and extreme depression. It will decrease strength, muscle mass, and bone mineral density. This could result in developing osteoporosis. It can plummet a man's energy level and drive in accomplishing daily activities. It can also create brain fog and a lack of focus. However, there is an answer to helping all of these symptoms. Testosterone replacement therapy is always an option, but long-term use does present health risks. However, a healthy diet and nutrition, as well as maintaining an active lifestyle can significantly improve these symptoms and keep your testosterone levels active and healthy. There are many other natural ways for a man to boost his testosterone levels naturally, but we will dive deeper into that later (Rush 2021).

In both male and female seniors, thyroid hormone imbalances can be a major disruption to their health. Remember, the thyroid is a small gland in the front of your neck. It controls the hormones produced to regulate body temperature, muscle strength, and metabolism. Both men and women over the age of sixty are at a higher risk for developing thyroid disease, which can result in weight gain, loss of strength, and hot flashes. However, there are ways to prevent and manage thyroid disease, including activity and diet (Rush, 2021).

If it seems like diet, nutrition, and activity are redundant in this chapter, that's because they are. So many people do not understand the significance our food, lifestyle, and habits have on our health. The natural ways to balance our hormones are directly correlated to how we live and what we eat. It is not crazy to believe that our systems rely on fuel. The truth is, while the medicine is absolutely necessary, it is not always the answer. And while most would have you believe that there is a pill for everything, sometimes it's better to get our health back the right way, instead of just covering up symptoms. Vitamins, supplements, and knowing the properties of the food you eat are some of the things we will start to take a look at. Because every plant has a purpose in the same way that every chemical in our body has a function.

So, age does play a role in our hormonal health and the way we develop, and everyone can, of all ages, experience a hormonal imbalance. There are many signs and side effects of someone going through a hormonal imbalance, and many risks involved, as well. But this does not mean there isn't hope, and these are things we must learn to live with. Like we said in the beginning, there are many ways to get our health and life back, we just have to navigate the murky waters of hormonal imbalance. So, let's continue on and look at the best avenues to take, if medication is the answer, and how to live again!

Chapter Summary

+ It's important to understand the differences between hormone imbalances in men and women.

+ Although it's normal for adolescence to go through puberty, they can still suffer from hormonal imbalances.

+ Identifying what a hormone imbalance looks like in a teenager is key to their growth and development.

+ Aging does not have to mean loss of energy, sexual function, and quality of life.

+ There are great ways to counteract the hormone imbalances that come with aging.

In the next chapter, you will learn….

+ Learn the differences between how hormone replacement and supplements affect our bodies.

+ Identify the side effects and possible dangers of hormone replacement.

+ Learn the natural supplements, their ingredients, and how they help hormone imbalances.

ALL NATURAL
ARE PRESCRIPTION HORMONES
THE ONLY ANSWER?

"Good nutrition creates health in all areas of our existence. All paths are interconnected." -T. Collin Campbell

Now that we have covered the ins and outs of hormonal imbalances, we are going to start looking at real solutions to help us manage these imbalances. We are going to look at how hormone medication operates and affects the body. We will also be looking at whether or not supplements, how they work, and if they are trustworthy or not. There are so many different options for hormonal imbalances, and it can be difficult to know the right path to take. Everyone has a different opinion and what someone should do when facing a hormonal imbalance, but ultimately, the right decision for you should be what works for your body and your health.

Let's start with the most common and most used form of hormone balancing pill out there: birth control. What is birth control? How does it work? Birth control was invented as a form of contraception for women. Once widely controversial, it is now more than accepted by society and used more than any other form of contraception available. However, birth control is prescribed to help manage a lot of other conditions and symptoms, as well. There are two types of oral birth control. One is a combination of both estrogen and progestin, and the other is strictly progestin. The combination pill works by halting ovulation and changing the lining of the uterus to keep sperm from attaching to an egg. Progestin, referred to as the "minipill," works by changing the consistency of mucus in the cervix by making it thicker, and occasionally stops ovulation (Cleveland Clinic, 2020).

While hormonal birth control is used for contraception, it can also be used to help regulate hormonal imbalances. Hormonal birth control can help to regulate and lighten menstruation, help and prevent anemia, improve bad acne, reduce chronic migraines, and manage PMS symptoms (Cleveland Clinic, 2020). While there are some cases that these hormones are absolutely beneficial and necessary, there are a lot of cases that can be remedied naturally instead of getting on hormonal birth control. Because while hormonal birth control can be helpful, it can also be harmful. First, hormonal birth control works by stopping a natural process in a woman's body. This can cause a lot of issues long-term, which most people don't talk about. Second, there are so many other symptoms that can accompany hormonal birth control, but we will get more into that later. Third, it can take up to three months for a woman to adjust to the hormones in oral birth control (Nurx, 2019). These are just a few of the glaring issues in birth control.

There are also many other forms of hormonal medications to help hormonal imbalances in women. For women experiencing vaginal dryness because of an imbalance in estrogen, there are vaginal estrogen creams that can be applied topically. There are also estrogen tablets and rings for people suffering from vaginal dryness. Eflornithine is also a prescription cream that can help halt facial hair growth in women (Medical News Today, 2021).

For men, hormone pills boil down to one hormone: testosterone. There is everything from testosterone pills to testosterone therapy. However, testosterone pills and therapy have less research behind them than hormonal birth control for women. There are a lot of benefits and side effects that can come with testosterone therapy. Overall, TRT is scientifically proven to be the best option for getting back normal testosterone levels. To young men suffering from an unusual hormonal imbalance, however, it might not be. So what is testosterone therapy and how does it work?

TRT stands for testosterone replacement therapy, and it is mainly used to treat low levels of testosterone that can hit men while they age. However, it's become mainstream for young men to boost their energy, sexual performance, and muscle mass. There are many forms of TRT and how it can be administered. There are also numerous ways TRT can be administered. If you are prescribed oral medication or topical cream, these need to be taken or applied daily. Intramuscular injections are the most effective. They allow the muscles to absorb the testosterone into the bloodstream quickly (Healthline, 2021). There are also other hormonal medications for both genders that can help with hormonal imbalances. Levothyroxine is a medication used to help with the symptoms of hypothyroidism. Metformin helps regulate low blood sugar levels for people with type two diabetes (Medical News Today, 2021). There are a lot of medications and treatments for hormonal imbalances, but are they the only answer? Let's flip the script. Take a look at supplements and how they work.

Supplements to balance aren't always cut and dry. Unlike medication, there is no "one-size-fits-all" pill that can cover up the symptoms of a hormonal imbalance. In so many cases, we see people suffering from all ailments, not just hormonal imbalances. They get prescribed medication that masks symptoms. This has become an epidemic in our culture. However, in recent years, focus on our health has differed from going to the doctor to receive a prescription for an ailment to discovering overall, bodily wellness. This means understanding our bodies and the way our systems work. With supplements, treatment is often a plan and a different lifestyle one has to embark on.

One of the great benefits of using supplements and nutrition for balancing hormonal imbalances is that there are so many "tools" one has when combining both. Herbs are a natural and gentle way to treat hormonal imbalance with no serious side effects or long-term impacts. It's also a great way to understand your bio-individuality and what your system needs in order to stay healthy. Medication is effective, but it does not truly grasp bio-individuality. Because everyone is different and has different levels of hormones, a prescribed medication could be the same for a 180-pound man as a 120-pound woman. With supplements, we find that there is often a nutrition plan that comes with it, and it is tapered to fit the individual person. Let's look at some great supplements used in treating hormone imbalances.

This first one is a great hormonal balancer for estrogen in women, or any man suffering from too high testosterone levels. Diindolylmethane, also known as DIM, is found in our cruciferous vegetables, otherwise known as leafy greens. Vegetables such as cabbage, kale, and broccoli contain high quantities of DIM. What is so crucial about these vegetables is the process it triggers after we eat it. According to Complete Care, after we eat vegetables like this, there is a precursor called indole-3-carbinol, which then is broken down into DIM during the digestion process (Complete Care, 2019).

Okay great, but what is so important about DIM? DIM has a large quantity of healing and balancing properties! First, it majorly supports the breakdown of estrogen in your liver, into healthy metabolites. Second, it prevents aromatase, which is the enzyme in charge of turning testosterone into estrogen. It also blocks a lot of the effects of testosterone and supports the cleansing and detox process of a cellular level, known as cellular detoxification. In a recent study, "DIM has shown chemopreventive activity during all stages of breast carcinogenesis," (Complete Care, 2019). DIM also can provide neuroprotection to help brain fog and prevent dementia, regulate your metabolism to prevent obesity, and reduce inflammation all over your body! It will regulate your estrogen levels but raise the good ones and lower the bad, while also inhibiting testosterone. There are many supplements of DIM, and it is recommended to take 100mg daily, before a meal (Complete Care, 2019).

The next supplements we are going to look at are really just herbs. However, these herbs are crucial for your liver function and detox process. A lot of our hormones are broken down and metabolized through our liver. If our liver is not functioning properly, hormones can build up and become toxic rather fast. This is why liver health is vital to achieving hormonal balance. Burdock and Dandelion Root both help in metabolizing and supporting your liver, and will help your hormones metabolize correctly as well (Burke, 2021).

This next supplement is wonderful for women suffering from bad, premenstrual syndrome. Vitex agnus-castus or chasteberry is a tree found in the Mediterranean. Recent studies found chasteberry to be helpful in boosting mood from hormonal depression, ease period cramps, and lower stress levels, which in turn can lower cortisol levels. It has also been proven to have properties that can boost hormone levels which can deplete with aging (Complete Care, 2019).

Lepidium Meyenii, or Maca, is a great overall balance of hormones as well as fertility. Maca grows in the highland regions of Peru at elevations between 14,000 to 16,000 feet (Complete Care 2019). It is an herbaceous plant that can be eaten raw, cooked, or ground into flour. It can be beneficial in all types of hormonal imbalances! Maca root has proven to boost serum levels in the luteinizing hormone, which is the hormone that supports fertility. According to Complete Care, "A study of nine men given 1500-3000mg of maca root daily for four months found that in increased seminal volume, sperm count, motile sperm count, and sperm motility, but did not alter their hormone levels," (Complete Care, 2019). During another study conducted, a group of men were given the same amount of maca for three months, and found their libido dramatically increased around month two!

Maca is also great for women going through the process of menopause. It can boost the function of the hypothalamus, pituitary glands, and gonadal glands, which are all a part of the reproductive axis. This can help alleviate hot flashes and vaginal dryness. Maca helps support bone density, preventing osteoporosis, which is common in pre-menopausal women. Studies have also shown that maca root can regulate blood sugar levels, stabilize mood, reduce anxiety, and boost energy (Complete Care, 2021). Maca root is a fantastic hormone balancer and fertility supporter. The average dose is between 1500-3000mg once a day.

Let's look at a few more vitamins and supplements which can greatly improve hormonal and all-over health. Ascorbic Acid or, Vitamin C, is essential for our neurotransmitters, antioxidants, tissue repair, and so much more. Vitamin C is a naturally occurring vitamin already in our systems, however, can easily become depleted leaving your body with a vitamin C deficiency. Because vitamin C is a major player in our cortisol hormone production, a person is more susceptible to a vitamin C deficiency during times of high stress. Taking a daily vitamin C supplement can reduce those cortisol levels and balance your adrenalin. Vitamin C is also key in lowering inflammation in your joints and muscles and boosting your immune system. It can also help the neurotransmitters in your brain balance, reducing chronic anxiety and depression. Studies have shown that Vitamin C has greatly helped women facing fertility issues, being a supporting role in restoring a healthy cycle and fertility (Complete Care, 2021).

Vitamin C also benefits our blood flow, because it works with our blood cells to support the cardiac output of blood flow to all of our organs. This is great for postmenopausal women who are struggling with low estrogen. For those with diabetes, vitamin C can help regulate fasting glucose, minimizing the effects of low or high blood sugar in the morning. Studies have shown that those taking daily vitamin C supplements had a twenty percent, all-cause, mortality rate than those who didn't, and that vitamin C reduced the risk of cancer in adult males. The recommended dose of vitamin C for an adult is about sixty milligrams a day. However, there is no harm in taking more. In fact, supplements with a higher dosage of vitamin C are often more beneficial than those with just sixty milligrams (Complete Care, 2021).

Everyone has seen those feel-good commercials promoting a probiotic as a cure-all at some point in their life. But what are probiotics really? And are they as beneficial as they say? Well, simply put, probiotics are good bacteria that already occur in our digestive tract. They make up the majority of the microbiome in our stomach. We know that the health of these microbiomes is extremely important, which makes probiotics extremely important, as well. An unhealthy microbiome can have a negative impact on your neurotransmitters (in both your stomach and your brain), digestion, and metabolism. Things like poor diet and nutrition, antibiotics, and chronic inflammation can hurt the natural probiotics in your gut (Complete Care, 2021).

So, yes probiotics are essential to our hormonal and overall health. While antibiotics are extremely necessary, modern medicine has taken antibiotic use to an extreme level. Avoiding using antibiotics unless absolutely necessary can help your probiotics produce and repopulate. A healthy diet and probiotic supplements are also key if you are struggling with depleted probiotics. See, probiotics help balance the production of serotonin in your brain, and an overgrowth of harmful bacteria, such as candida (or yeast), can kill probiotics. This can lead to chronic yeast infections, weight gain, and depression. And this is just one example of a harmful bacteria that can kill our probiotics! Daily intake of probiotics can balance mood disorders like anxiety, depression, and bipolar disorder. According to Complete Care, "In healthy elderly adults, short-term probiotic supplementation can enhance immune function," (Complete Care, 2021). Finding the right probiotic supplement for your body is vital for your hormonal balance. A good probiotic will have a large range of different bacteria and will typically be refrigerated. If not, be sure to check that it's safe to take at room temperature (Complete Care, 2021).

The next two supplements enhance one another so we will look at them together. Vitamin B6 and magnesium are great hormonal stabilizers that tend to go hand-in-hand. If you have a deficiency in one, you probably are deficient in the other. Magnesium is a mineral, while B6 is a vitamin part of the vitamin B group. Both are vital for our natural nutrients and health. Magnesium plays an important role in our cortisol levels and the effects stress can have on our bodies. It also correlates with inflammation, heart rhythms, sleep patterns, and blood pressure. This is due to the fact that over three hundred enzymes in our bodies use magnesium to function properly (Complete Care, 2021).

Vitamin B6 is a water-soluble vitamin that has great effects on our energy levels and production. For vitamin B6, there are over one hundred enzymes that count vitamin B6 for our amino acids, metabolism, and glucose levels. Vitamin B6 can help with stress and anxiety levels, and for women, can greatly help with negative symptoms during PMS. Taking a magnesium and vitamin B supplement together can help each of them work better for your body. This is because they both help in a lot of the same functions and bounce off each other to stabilize hormones. An adult can take up to 2500 milligrams of magnesium a day and one to three milligrams of vitamin B6 (Complete Care, 2021).

Now, let's look at calcium and copper. Both are minerals that are important for our brain, cortisol, and bone health. Zinc is the second most abundant trace metal in humans next to iron (Complete Care, 2021). Just like magnesium, your body has over three hundred enzymes that rely on zinc in order to function. Some of those enzymes correlate to our neurotransmitters and the production and release of serotonin and cortisol. Zinc has been found to have a positive effect on mood and can prevent depression as well as help your body build resilience to stress. Premenopausal women should take zinc, as it can help balance the mood swings that come with it. It is also important for pregnant women to take zinc whether it be through supplementation or their diet. However, it's important to note that too much zinc can increase one's risk of heart disease, so consuming the correct amount for your age and weight is key (Complete Care, 2021). Be sure to consult a doctor or professional to find out how much zinc you should be consuming on a daily basis.

Copper is a diverse element that also plays a diverse role in our hormonal health. It supports the transportation of oxygen and our bodies also turn copper into an enzyme called superoxide. "Superoxide is a by-product of oxygen metabolism, and if not regulated, causes many types of cell damage," (Complete Care, 2021). This means that without copper, our superoxide dismutase can decrease, and free radicals can have free reign to hurt the cells in your body. Taking copper supplements can help with depression, decrease heart enlargement, and prevent osteoporosis. It will help prevent free radicals from damaging your cells and creating hormonal imbalances. A healthy, daily intake of copper is about one to one and a half milligrams (Complete

Care, 2021).

If that seems like a long list of supplements, you should know that there are so many more vitamins and minerals that can help in hormone health. But for now, it's a good start. After all of that, let's dive into the matter at hand: pills versus supplements. Please understand this is not a smear campaign against doctors or prescription medication. Prescription medication can be necessary and vital for certain hormonal imbalances and in all other aspects of health. There is no disputing that. However, there are many negative side effects that can come from hormone prescriptions, and this is simply a dive into what those look like. Some are short-term, but others are long-term.

While hormonal birth control is sometimes used to regulate hormones, oftentimes, it can have the opposite effect. Since hormonal birth control works by essentially stopping ovulation, it can take a toll on your hormone production. Women can experience a variety of symptoms such as extreme mood swings, irritability, headaches, weight fluctuation, nausea, tender breasts, and unscheduled bleeding. This is all due to the fact that their hormone production has been disrupted at a certain level, and while other symptoms may have disappeared, new ones have now presented themselves (Nurx, 2021). Then, there are the more serious, long-term effects of hormonal birth control.

Studies have shown that some women taking the combination pill have an increased risk for developing blood clots, stroke, heart attack, and high blood pressure (Cleveland Clinic, 2020).

In men, testosterone replacement therapy is the most popular form of "pill" for hormone imbalances. Studies have shown that TRT can be extremely beneficial for aging men who are experiencing the negative side effects of decreased testosterone. If done safely and by a professional with controlled, natural doses, TRT can improve energy, muscle mass, sex drive, and overall health (WebMD, 2020). However, TRT can also be abused and cause many negative side effects if not taken with caution. Young men who do not have a decrease in testosterone are more at risk to experience serious side effects of TRT. Short-term side effects can include infertility due to low sperm count, shrinkage of the testicles, and acne. Long-term side effects can include an increased risk of heart attacks, blood clots, and stroke (WebMD, 2020).

So, which route is better? Ultimately, that decision is up to you and what you feel is best for your body, but this book is about regaining our hormonal health naturally! This isn't to say that you should self-diagnose and begin taking supplements based on your own understanding. Having your blood levels read and diagnosed by a specialist is equally important when beginning supplements. In addition, your blood levels should be read on a consistent basis to ensure that the supplements you're taking are positively impacting your hormonal imbalance (Refinery, 2020). But supplements have fewer to no side effects in comparison to medication, and a well-balanced lifestyle and diet is a great starting point. The truth is that most of our vitamins and supplements should come through the nutrients in our diet, but supplements can be extremely beneficial in helping reverse and regulate hormonal imbalances.

The natural route is often the safest and most preventative way to combat hormonal imbalances. Like we mentioned earlier, birth control disrupts our natural hormones, thereby canceling out the natural hormonal imbalance. If our bodies are constantly fighting for homeostasis, how does disrupting the natural order of bodily functions help achieve hormonal balance? Band-aiding symptoms instead of healing the issue is only going to prolong the struggle. The bottom line is that most hormonal imbalances occur because our core nutrients, lifestyle, and diet are not beneficial for our bodies. Hormones respond to every single thing we put into our bodies. This isn't about having control over our hormones, it's about taking care of them. In the same way, you take care of your house, dogs, children, or work life, your body and hormones require the same amount of dedication in order to function properly. Healing your hormones naturally is more than just finding supplements. It's changing your diet and lifestyle to care for them too.

Chapter Summary

◆   Knowing how forms of hormonal birth control and TRT replacement work is important so you can make an informed decision for your health.

◆   Understanding the ingredients in different supplements and how they can benefit your body is important for making the correct supplement choice.

◆   Understanding the side effects hormone replacement can cause is vital in choosing the best route for you.

In the next chapter, you will learn….

◆   The importance of food and how different types can affect your body.

◆   The beginning stages of what a hormone-balancing diet can look like.

◆   How our culture has changed food and what it's doing to our overall health.

◆   An important list of things you should avoid as well as eat for your hormones.

THE DREADED DIET EATING FOR HORMONAL IMBALANCE

"Eating well is a form of self-respect." -Anonymous

We have looked at hormones, their functions, types of hormonal imbalances, and supplements that can help balance them. Now, we will embark on a journey into the key to all of our health and hormonal imbalances: diet. We have briefly mentioned the effects diet and poor nutrition can have on our hormones, but this chapter is going to dissect everything you think you know about diet. This isn't a fad diet to lose a few pounds. This isn't a short-term phase to fix your hormonal imbalance. This is a lifestyle choice, change, and beginning to a new future.

"Certain foods can help to restore balance while others can completely destroy it," (Rosenblum, 2021). This quote from Carlyn Rosenblum, founder of MTHR Nutrition, is extremely accurate when it comes to the correlation of diet to our hormones. We have learned that gut health is vital for our overall health, as well as hormone balance. This is because everything we consume is processed and placed through this intricate system. Therefore, the foods we choose to eat will play a major role in the response of our hormones. There are so many sources around us contributing to a hormonal imbalance, many of them you may have never thought of. Things like fertilizers sprayed on produce, meat is grown with chemical hormones, excess sugar intake, and excess dairy intake can all negatively impact our hormone health (Rosenblum, 2021).

For instance, chronic inflammation and high blood sugar can be directly correlated to food products. Alcohol, caffeine, and dairy can be the cause of these hormonal imbalances. There is a protein in dairy which can increase cortisol, which can then lead to chronic inflammation of the joints. Alcohol and caffeine can also increase cortisol which can cause a rise in blood pressure. If your blood sugar becomes chronically high, this can then trigger higher insulin production, which then raises your androgen levels (Rosenblum, 2021). Non-organic produce is sprayed with pesticides. Studies have shown the chemicals disrupt your endocrine system and contain artificial hormones, easily causing a hormonal imbalance (Rosenblum, 2021). See how everything in our bodies is connected, and it all begins with the food we choose to fuel it with.

We've talked about how important healthy fats are for our hormones, but did you know that they are essential for every single hormone production in our bodies? Fiber is also vital to our hormone health because it boosts gut health and binds to toxins and excess hormones to flush them out of our system. Antioxidants can reduce inflammation and cortisol, which can help manage stress and excess estrogen (Rosenblum, 2021).

So, what are some healthy foods to begin your diet? Let's start with healthy fats. Wild-caught salmon is a great source of protein. Wild-caught means it's not farm-raised, so the salmon only consumes what's in its natural environment. This is important because farm-raised salmon consume a forced diet that is made up of grains, corn, and fish oil. Secondly, salmon is high in Omega-3's. Avocados are another great option for a filling, healthy-fat snack. They contain high levels of monounsaturated fat (which simply means naturally occurring fat) and fiber. They can help increase hormone production and regulate blood sugar (Rosenblum, 2021).

Cruciferous vegetables, like kale, broccoli, and cauliflower, are high in antioxidants and fiber. This can play a major role in reducing high cortisol levels and also eliminate excess hormones. Another food, which is known as a 'superfood,' is flaxseed. Flaxseed is a natural anti-inflammatory and also has phytoestrogens. This can increase low estrogen levels occurring in women. Sweet potatoes are a healthy filler that helps your liver with the detoxification process. They also contain high levels of vitamin B6, fiber, and antioxidants. For all the plant-based eaters out there, two great plant-based proteins are lentils and spirulina. Spirulina contains antioxidants that aid in detoxifying your system and reducing stress (Rosenblum, 2021).

Proteins are tricky when it comes to balancing hormonal health because they are bio-individual. Certain proteins might work for one person, but not for another. See, when using proteins for hormonal balance, certain types of protein are going to help your specific imbalance more than others. However, good sources of protein are essential for hormonal health as they provide amino acids which are vital in the production of insulin, estrogen, and thyroid hormones (Gottfried, 2021).

Protein is bio-individual because everyone has a different blueprint to the way their hormones respond to outside stimuli. People with Celiac Disease or gluten intolerance may cause a hormonal imbalance by eating grain-fed beef, leading to poor gut health or 'leaky gut.' Proteins can also shift the microbiome in your gut, causing them to imbalance, specifically affecting estrogen levels. Legumes can trigger other individuals by overstimulating their immune systems and creating inflammation (Gottfried, 2021). This might seem like protein is not great for hormonal health, but remember, it also produces those necessary amino acids needed for estrogen, thyroid, and insulin hormones.

Women's hormonal responses to nutrition are always unique, especially when it comes to protein. Dr. Sara Gottfried found that "When women eat grain-fed, hormone-injected, superbug-infected meat, it can negatively impact digestion and may cause bloating and constipation," (Gottfried, 2021). This is a horribly negative effect on one's gut health, which can then lead to a rise in estrogen levels. While meat can contain healthy fats at a higher level than grains, legumes, or nuts, there is a larger societal issue with meat we are facing. It is the unprocessed, chemically produced materials that can be easily hidden in the fat of meat bought in a grocery store (Gottfried, 2021).

Our bodies are hard-wired for the "hunter-gatherer" diet. This dates back to ancient times when we had to constantly resource and hunt our own food for survival. Our bodies respond well to a high intake of vegetables, seeds, and nuts, fruit from time to time, and clean proteins. These are the natural things your body's hormones and overall health crave. Elevated levels of estrogen are more likely to occur when a woman is eating processed, conventionally raised, red meat. A heavy meat diet also ups the risk for obesity and studies have linked it to a higher body mass index and larger waist in women. Eating a more plant-based diet with natural, lean proteins has proven to lead to regular estrogen levels. This is due to the fact that your diet contains more fiber which aids in the removal of excess estrogen (Gottfried, 2021).

Protein's effect on the thyroid hormone is also something to be cautious of when selecting the proteins which are right for you. The biggest player in thyroid imbalances is protein sources with the gluten additive. In fact, one of the leading causes of hypothyroidism is autoimmune thyroiditis. This occurs through our gut, and when gluten enters our gut, it can attach itself to the microbiome lining our intestines and begin to kill it, leading to autoimmune thyroiditis. People with Celiac Disease have a higher risk of developing these conditions (Gottfried, 2021).

Mercury found in fish can also lead to thyroid

hormone imbalances. High mercury disrupts your endocrine system, upsetting the balance of both your thyroid and estrogen. Individuals with a high-mercury diet put themselves at risk for developing mercury toxicity and thyroid disorders. This is because mercury and iodine appear similar in the human body, and our bodies will store mercury in place of iodine. We need iodine to help regulate our body's detoxification process (Gottfried, 2021).

Protein can hurt the balance of insulin, as well. Because we rely on fiber to help stabilize our blood sugar and prevent diabetes, relying on a protein-heavy diet decreases your fiber intake and can hurt your insulin balance. There are new, emerging studies that have shown a plant-based diet has more advantages over our insulin and glucose balance. According to Dr. Sara Gottfried, "A Paleo-based food plan helps improve blood sugars in the short-term, and the much more sustainable Mediterranean diet (low in meat in general but does feature seafood and other lean proteins) has a wealth of research supporting its role in preventing mitigating type two diabetes," (Gottfried, 2021). While protein is essential for our health, it is key to understand the type of protein your body requires, as well as what is in the protein you consume. Just like with everything else, unnatural, chemically processed meat will only wreak havoc on your hormones.

Now, let's take a closer look at all the true, good foods. Living in a society where food has become a form of entertainment but lost a lot of its nutritional purpose, it can seem like an overwhelming task trying to figure out the right foods to eat. Earlier in the chapter, we briefly mentioned a few great sources of good foods, but there are so many more. First, organic vegetables and fruits are excellent for achieving and maintaining hormone balance. Monitoring your protein intake is key as well, and be sure to make sure it is full of lean protein. These can include wild-caught fish, chicken breasts, grass-fed beef, eggs, lentils, and nuts. Fruits are a great source of energy and natural sugar. Leafy greens such as kale, spinach, broccoli, and cauliflower are essential for your nutritional health and great foods to eat. Good sources of healthy fats like avocados, olive oil, coconut oil, tree nuts, and organic butter (yes, butter), are good foods.

If you think butter being a good food sounds crazy, you're not alone. As a collective, we have avoided butter as most people associate it with bad cholesterol and overall heart health. However, organic natural butter is whipped, which eliminates those bad enzymes we went over previously. Butter, when mixed with bleached, wheat flour, or processed sugars is bad. But when it stands alone or is used in conjunction with healthy foods, it can be a great source of energy and helpful, healthy fat. Other good foods you should incorporate are functional carbs such as rice, quinoa, sweet potatoes, yams, and whole grains (if you do not have a sensitivity to gluten). Chia seeds and flaxseeds are fantastic sources of fiber and antioxidants that can also be a filling snack throughout your day (Pagán, 2021).

There are also some great daily routines you can implement beginning your lifestyle change. Digestion plays a key role in our gut health, and a great way to wake it up is doing a shot of apple cider vinegar and water when you first wake up. Apple cider vinegar can also help restore the microbiome lining your intestines and also metabolize fat. Enjoying ginger, spearmint, or lemon tea in the morning can also be super beneficial to restoring gut health. Lastly, keeping your plate balanced is a great way to ensure you are getting adequate nutrients to combat hormonal imbalances. With every meal, your plate should be divided into one-half leafy greens, one-fourth lean, healthy protein, and one-fourth nutritional crabs like rice or quinoa (Bhatia, 2020).

Now, for the hard part - the bad foods. Let's start with the most obvious, which is sugar. Processed sugars, specifically, can spike your insulin and can also transfer sugar from your bloodstream directly into your cells. Processed sugars such as candy, soda, pastries, ice cream, or anything product containing high processed sugars should be avoided. Not to say these cannot be enjoyed from time to time, but they should not be a part of your regular diet. When processed sugar is consumed regularly, your body focuses more on processing insulin and will neglect other vital hormones (Moody, 2019).

Another hard fact we have to face is the truth about bread. Bread, especially white bread, can cause a variety of issues for your hormone health. What most people don't realize is that gluten can have a negative impact on everyone, not just those with Celiac Disease or gluten sensitivities. See, back in the 1940s scientists realized that by increasing the gluten protein found in wheat products, they could extend the shelf-life of these products by three weeks, therefore monopolizing the wheat industry. The wheat products we consume today are not made with natural chemicals. The gluten today increases all-over inflammation in the body, significantly stresses the adrenal glands and thyroid glands, and attacks our immune system. Wheat and gluten products can lead to a decreased production of hormones from your thyroid, adrenals, and gonads (Moody, 2019).

Dairy is another production to avoid when balancing your hormones. First of all, any non-organic dairy is full of growth hormones and antibiotic residue. Second, the enzymes in dairy are made to nurture calves in the same way that breast milk is made to nurture human babies. So, cow's milk can be very hard on our digestive system and cause inflammation, especially in the sinus cavities. This can lead to chronic bad allergies and sinus infections. Dairy can also cause inflammation and build-up in your skin, leading to bad acne (Moody 2019).

Two more things you will need to avoid or minimize intake are caffeine and alcohol. Alcohol interferes with a lot of our hormone production. First, alcohol is metabolized as sugar in our bloodstream. This can mess with insulin levels. It also disrupts your hypothalamus and pituitary gland. These are what send messages to your brain and body of what hormones you need. Alcohol can also trigger cortisol, and decrease testosterone. Too much caffeine will disrupt your sleep cycle, causing cortisol levels to increase, as well (Moody, 2019). This isn't to say you can't have a drink every now and then or enjoy a cup of coffee in the morning. But both of these things should be heavily monitored and limited in order to achieve hormone balance.

Nightshades are another food group that should be limited. Now, nightshades are a family of flowering plants that contain chemical compounds called alkaloids. Vegetables such as tomatoes, white potatoes, eggplants, bell peppers, and spices sourced from peppers (not including black pepper), are all nightshades. In large, concentrated quantities, alkaloids are poisonous. Concentrated amounts of nightshade are used to make nerve gas! But don't worry, these vegetables only contain a low amount of nightshade and won't cause nerve damage to the human body. However, when dealing with a hormonal imbalance, it's important to limit your intake of nightshades, as they can cause inflammation all over our system (Moody, 2019).

Some other foods to avoid include high-fructose corn syrup, packaged fried snacks, and artificial sweeteners. High-fructose corn syrup found in most processed foods decreases leptin which is the hormone that tells our body when we are full. This can lead to overeating resulting in weight gain. Packaged fried foods contain high levels of trans fat, which can hinder testicular function in men and lower testosterone levels. Artificial sweeteners hurt the probiotics in your intestines and can lower your levels of hunger hormones (Greatest, 2021). This probably feels like a long list of foods to avoid, but when you swap them out for the good foods, your life will ultimately change, and you won't feel like you're missing out on anything.

We've all known water is vital to our survival and we've all been lectured on the importance of daily water intake. However, water is critical for getting hormones back to homeostasis and keeping them that way. Our tissues and organs function under specific biochemical and hormonal conditions, and any outside factor that compromises those conditions can wreck our system. "Water is the most refreshing and revitalizing solvent that has the capacity to dissolve and remove impurities from the blood," (Dr. Elist, 2021). Even tiny changes in the hydration of our tissues can affect our hormonal systems, the process of nutrients, and the concentration of toxins. Let's look at two functions that can be hurt from poor water intake.

First, tissue hydration plays a major role in the breakdown of our hormones. If we are not consuming the correct intake of water, our tissues cannot break down the old hormones and circulate the new, functioning ones. This can lead to a toxic level of hormonal buildup. Second, the blood supply to our liver and kidneys can be hindered when our water intake is consistently low. And we know that almost all of our hormones are metabolized in the liver and released through the kidneys. If either one of these organs is not receiving an adequate blood supply, our hormones and metabolism will be affected directly (Dr. Elist, 2021).

Increasing your water intake can also be the most efficient solution to hormonal imbalances that come with the aging process. Drinking more water has proven to support skin, hair, nails, bladder irritation, brain function, and ease symptoms of menopause for women. According to Dr. Lisa Moscone, "Eighty percent of the brain's content is water. And every single chemical reaction that happens in the brain needs water to occur, including energy production.

So, if you don't have enough, your brain will just not be able to make energy," (Gennev, 2021). It's not just about the loss of energy, though. Water is so critical to our hormonal health that even a two percent decrease in water intake can leave the brain with confusion, brain fog, and extreme fatigue. Any decrease in water could also cause dry skin, brittle hair and nails, headaches, bloating, and constipation (Gennev, 2021). Water is one of the most important things to increase and keep track of in order to achieve hormonal balance!

Overall, diet is more than dieting, it's changing the way you perceive food as a whole. Food is essential for every aspect of our health, and the cultural shift of viewing food as entertainment has completely wrecked our health. The idea that food is entertainment and prescriptions are the answer to every issue, has become normalized. This is like reading half of the book and writing a paper about the ending. Yes, prescriptions and medications are absolutely necessary in some cases. But if we want to achieve hormonal balance and reclaim our health, we need to start reading the whole book. This means getting to know our bio-individuality, becoming conscious of food and its properties, and looking at food as a medicine too.

Chapter Summary

- Specific foods can lead to chronic inflammation and stress which can then lead to hormonal imbalance.
- Certain foods like cruciferous vegetables and healthy fats promote hormone balance.
- Even a slight decrease in hydration can lead to numerous hormone imbalances.
- Water and the foods we eat are crucial to our health and hormone happiness.

In the next chapter, you will learn….
- What working out really means and if you really have to join a gym to maintain a healthy life.
- Great, practical ways to stay consistent with physical activity.
- Other, small techniques to balance your stress levels and hormones.

RUN FOR THE HILLS
HOW EXERCISE HELPS YOUR
HORMONES

"In today's fast-paced, technology-driven society, it is more important than ever to make time to exercise. Exercise is a productive outlet that stimulates feel-good transmitters that help boost overall well-being," -Hahns Petty.

Probably even more dreaded than diet, is regular exercise. However, exercising regularly is key to attaining hormonal balance and overall health. It can greatly reduce issues like stress, anxiety, weight gain, and insomnia. Before you run from this chapter (no pun intended) let's get one thing straight. Exercising regularly does not necessarily mean joining a gym. Anyone can exercise at home, outside, or anywhere. This chapter is going to focus on the benefits of staying active, how different types of exercise affect your hormones and finding the best routine for you. For some, the gym provides release. For others, the gym is a torture chamber. Whichever category you land in, is absolutely okay. But regular exercise and activity are important for our hormones, so let's dive into some great exercises that can be done anywhere.

Since a workout routine is preference-based, there are many types of workouts you can do from home. Some prefer a gym or fitness club because it keeps them motivated to continue. However, others find the solace of their own home better for achieving a great workout. First, there are hundreds of fantastic apps and in-home workout plans right at your fingertips. These typically come with a coach or tracker to help you stay on top of a weekly routine. If you love running, this can be done by hitting the sidewalks or trails right outside of your home. Buying a set of dumbbells to incorporate into your workout routine is beneficial as well. Workouts like push-ups, air squats, burpees, and ab routines all keep you active and can be achieved from home. In-home partner workouts can also be a great way to keep you motivated and on track!

But what does regular exercise do for our hormones? First of all, exercise positively impacts many hormones in our body, specifically your "feel good" hormones. Studies have shown that dopamine and serotonin are directly affected by physical activity. Exercise increases dopamine levels which in turn help decrease cortisol levels. This can lower stress and the effects it has on the body. An increase in dopamine can also help regulate mood swings and irritability. Regular exercise also releases the hormone serotonin. This can be extremely beneficial for individuals who suffer from insomnia and sleep apnea. A boost in serotonin can also help with depression and anxiety, appetite, memory and sexual function, and social anxiety (Piedmont Healthcare, 2021).

Dopamine and serotonin aren't the only two hormones that exercise can enhance. Testosterone and estrogen positively respond to regular exercise as well. Physical activity can drastically boost testosterone levels in men. This is important, especially as men age. Regularly engaging in exercise can slow the loss of testosterone as a man gets older. Studies also show that regular physical activity increases estrogen levels in women. This is specifically great for combating menopause symptoms in women over the age of fifty (Piedmont Healthcare, 2021).

There are certain types of different exercises that can specifically benefit hormonal health. HIIT is a type of training that targets your cardiovascular response in order to burn more calories. HIIT stands for high-intensity interval training. It is comprised of intense exercise in short bursts, followed by a quick period of rest. HIIT has proven to burn more fat than aerobic exercise and it can increase the human growth hormone (HGH). HGH improves metabolism, muscle growth, and recovery. HGH can manage insulin sensitivity, which can be beneficial in managing conditions like diabetes and heart disease. It can also help you lose weight (Basile, 2021).

Yoga and Pilates are two more types of exercise that can greatly improve hormone health. The stretching and deep breathing involved in yoga can be an excellent balancer for your cortisol levels, as it reduces stress. Pilates and yoga are both great mood stabilizers and can be especially beneficial for women going through menopause. However, while these are great for balancing hormones, really any type of exercise is good for them too. 10,000 steps a day is a great goal to try to hit as often as you can. Physical activity can truly change the course of your hormonal imbalance (Basile, 2021).

Getting into a new exercise routine can be difficult, to say the least. Staying consistent with working out is the main problem most people face. It's easy to let life, stress, and other factors get in the way of working out. If we throw in a hormonal imbalance, there's another factor that makes consistent working out feel like an impossible task. Chronic inflammation can make actual exercise painful and demotivating. But don't lose heart! There are numerous ways to make working out a normal part of your daily routine.

First, one instrumental thing to know is that it takes three weeks or twenty-one days for our bodies to adjust to something new. If you can get through three weeks of consistently working out, it will stop feeling like a task and begin to feel like a normal part of your daily routine. The key is to do a type of exercise that works for you. Next, treat it like your job. You show up for your job, every day because your livelihood depends on it. In the same way, your health depends on your exercise, so you must show up! Some people prefer to work out first thing in the morning. This gets it out of the way for the day, and sets your hormone levels in balance, and makes you feel good for the rest of what you have planned. However, working out when best fits in your schedule is an important factor in making it a consistent occurrence (Basile, 2021).

Another great way to jump into the habit of working out is to make it a fun activity that you genuinely enjoy! It doesn't just have to be a task that you struggle through. If working out bores you, you are more likely to not stick with it. If you love running, get up early and hit the trails while listening to your favorite music. If you love to dance, throw some strength training into a fun dance routine. Keeping yourself engaged is the best way to stay consistent with working out (Basile, 2021).

Now, let's talk about stretching. We all know that warming up is important before you work out, but what about after? First, warming up is very important to prevent injuries. Think of your muscles like a rubber band. They stretch and grow depending on what you do with them. Now, what if you stick that rubber band in the freezer and then try to use it? It breaks. Stretching or working out when your muscles are cold can be dangerous and put you at higher risk to sustain energy. It's extremely important to warm up before you work out, and stretch after. Warm-up by walking on an incline or doing anything that gets your blood flowing. Your muscles respond much better to stretching when they are warm. They become more pliable and we are able to push them a bit farther than we could if we were cold.

Having an accountability partner can also be an ideal way to make working out a normal habit. First, it becomes a goal and activity to do with a friend or partner. Second, reporting back to someone on your workouts will make you more inclined to do them. Working out can seem like a daunting task, but remember that you are doing this for yourself. Changing your perspective from "getting through a workout" to a way you are caring for yourself can take the pressure off and make it an easier thing to integrate into your day. Whatever type of physical activity you choose, it should be because you genuinely love and desire to take care of your body. You're reading this because you want to reclaim your health, and working out is a simple step in that process.

Now, let's take a look at anaerobic and aerobic exercise. Anaerobic exercise means that this type of exercise doesn't force your body to use oxygen. Anaerobic exercise breaks down the glucose that's already in your muscles for energy. Strength training and HIIT are examples of anaerobic exercise. Aerobic exercise means that your body uses oxygen for energy while working out. Any type of cardio such as running, biking, and swimming are all examples of this. Since both types affect the body in different ways, let's take a look at both of them and see the benefits and pitfalls that come with each.

Anaerobic exercise can be extremely beneficial to your hormonal health. It raises your heart rate in short intervals and gives room for short rest in-between. The reason anaerobic exercise is done in short intervals is that our bodies can't handle long periods of these types of exercises. According to Craig Ehleider, president of Kennedy Fitness,

"Anaerobic exercise is not only used for strength training, but for those who want to harden their bones and muscles, which is important to do as we age," (Jefferson Health, 2021). Anaerobic exercise increases the human growth hormone more than aerobic exercise. HGH boosts your metabolism, strengthens bones, and builds muscle. Certain studies have shown men benefit more from anaerobic exercise due to their higher testosterone level which supports HGH, but this is not to say women can't benefit from it as well. If you are wanting to begin this type of exercise, it's important to ease into it. Finding a professional trainer can be a great starting point, but light weights and easy workouts can also be a starting point (Jefferson Health, 2021).

Stress, smoking, and alcohol can trigger our bodies into thinking we are in danger, sending our hormones into fight or flight mode. This means our adrenaline and cortisol levels rapidly increase and cause damage to our systems. Weight gain, weak immune systems, high blood pressure, and weight gain can all occur from this rise in hormones. Because anaerobic exercise increases your HGH, it can combat the increased adrenaline and cortisol levels. Anaerobic secrets more HGH than any other type of exercise (Jefferson Health, 2021).

Aerobic exercise, or cardio, is beneficial for many

aspects of your health. First, cardio is amazing at countering the effects of depression and mood swings. Aerobic exercise brings a sense of exhilaration during, with a calm wave following. It can greatly benefit anxiety and other types of mood disorders, as well. But how exactly does cardio help things like depression and anxiety? According to Harvard Medical School, "The mental benefits of aerobic exercise have a neurochemical basis. Exercise reduces the levels of the body's stress hormones, such as adrenaline and cortisol. It also stimulates the production of endorphins," (Harvard Medical, 2021). Have you ever experienced or heard someone talk about a "runner's high?" This is the endorphins releasing during the run, setting off an almost euphoric feeling (Harvard Medical, 2021).

Everyone has different opinions on which type of exercise is better for your health, but keeping a balance of both is best to balance hormones. With anaerobic exercise, the more intense a workout, the more hormones are secreted. Aerobic exercise steadily releases small amounts of hormones over a certain period of time. There is no style of workout that is better for you, as long as you are careful and keep the proper form with whatever it is you're doing.

The truth is that all exercise can have neurological, emotional, hormonal, and behavioral benefits. Exercise is one of the best things you can do for your mental health.

Whether it's a runner's high, great lift, or relaxing yoga class, the sense of accomplishment which follows boosts serotonin levels in your brain. With consistent working outcomes a sense of control, self-confidence, and a better self-image. Please don't misunderstand. Self-confidence isn't just from the weight loss benefit of working out. The physical act of committing to improvement and following through gives you more confidence than your body image ever will.

Exercise can also be used as an escape when you are stressed. Whether you enjoy working out in a group setting or in solidarity, the act of taking some time out of your day to focus on your physical health renews your energy and drive. Exercise should be something you look forward to - a recreational act that gets you out and moving. When you're focused on working out, everything else melts away. This gives your brain a rest from the stressors of the day, and allows space for creativity and fun. Even going on a twenty-minute walk can relieve stress and clear your head.

Because stress is often a part of our daily lives and there are so many imbalances and symptoms that follow, working out has become an outlet for most people. So, let's take a look at a few more types of exercises that can be beneficial in reducing stress. We know how stress affects our hormones and the symptoms accompanying it, but chronic stress can also result in muscle tissues as well. Taut facial expressions and constant clenching of the jaw can result in severe jaw pain which leads to chronic headaches. Tense muscles often lead to an aching back and shoulders. While physical fitness benefits stress, sometimes, when our body isn't performing the way we want it to, it can easily turn into another stressful situation. "Autoregulation exercises are techniques created to replace the spiral of stress with a cycle of response," (Harvard Health, 2021). What does this mean? Basically, autoregulation is adjusting your workload and intensity of every workout, based on your performance in the previous one.

For example, if your body isn't responding as strongly as it did in your last workout, it might mean you need to lower the intensity and resistance of your session. This might sound strange, as most people feel the need to push themselves in a workout. But consistently working out means burnout, both physical and mental, is a possibility. Depending on your day, nutrient and water intake, and environmental factors, your body will respond to physical activity differently. You're not going to improve and feel amazing during every single workout. Using autoregulation to track your workouts can help you see how far you've come and prevented you from pushing too hard on days your body isn't ready (Harvard Health, 2021).

Breathing exercises are another way to manage stress and hormone levels. While they are commonly associated with yoga, stand-alone breathing exercises are also an option. Breathing correctly is not something we typically think about on a day-to-day basis. When breathing deeply, think of pushing your stomach out as you intake air. The "square" breathing technique is used in meditation and stress relief. It works like this. First, picture the outline of a square, then on the inhale follow one side of the square down for five seconds. Next, hold that breath along the bottom of the square for five seconds. Exhale following the other side of the square up for five seconds, and holding again on the top of the square for another five seconds. You can do this wherever and whenever you need. Doing this throughout your day has proven to prevent increased cortisol levels that come from stress, especially if you do this over six times a day (Harvard Medical, 2021).

We've focused on how much physical exercise can benefit our hormones and health, but what about mental exercise? Mental exercise is just as important for our hormones as physical. This doesn't mean downloading a brain app or working crossword puzzles. Mental exercise can range from journaling your thoughts to talking about your problems with a friend or therapist. Meditation is also a great way to exercise your mind. Mental stress speeds up our heart rate and blood flow, which can raise your blood pressure. Studies have shown that meditation can, "slow the heart rate, lower the blood pressure, reduce the rapid breathing rate, diminish the body's oxygen consumption, reduce blood adrenaline levels, and change skin temperature," (Harvard Health, 2021). All of this can give our body a relaxation response, therefore lowering cortisol and stress levels. The best way to meditate is to set aside a select time everyday so you can stay committed to it. Also, be sure the time you meditate is free of outside distractions and in a place that makes you feel calm. Lightening is key and low-lighting is best to create a calm atmosphere (Harvard Health, 2021).

Just like in our diets, this is about exercise is more than a phase or short-term solution. Making exercise a part of your lifestyle will change the course of your hormone health. Taking care of yourself and your hormones is bigger than dieting and exercising for a short amount of time. It's about changing the way you live, think, and act. Exercise is not only about changing our physical appearance. While changing your physical appearance by working out can increase your mood and serotonin levels, it is too often the sole reason people want to start working out. This can often create a counterproductive system. When one doesn't see physical results as soon they want, it can be disheartening, causing a lack of motivation to set in. Working out might fall to the wayside, as results were not what they wanted. However, you cannot see what's changing on the inside. Your physical appearance will change in time, but the inward benefits will begin to happen almost immediately.

The drive to work out should come from the realization that you deserve a healthy life, which means you deserve to take care of yourself. You are worth the time and effort changing your lifestyle will take. You deserve to set aside time to focus on your health and well-being. You deserve to buy healthy and delicious food in order to get your hormones back in balance. You deserve hormonal balance.

Chapter Summary

*   Working out looks different for everyone and you don't need to join a gym to stay healthy.
*   How hormones affect dopamine and serotonin levels to promote a healthy and balanced hormonal system.
*   How exercise affects our mental health and stress levels and can bring us back to center.
*   How various breathing techniques can settle digestion, stress, and sleep patterns.

In the next chapter, you will learn….
*   What changing your life really means.
*   Practical ways to change your lifestyle and promote healthy hormones.
*   How to manage these lifestyle changes and start down the path to a healthier life.

LIVING THE LIFE
LIFESTYLE ADJUSTMENTS FOR HORMONAL BALANCE

"We cannot become what we want by remaining what we are," -Max Depree.

Now, let's map out that healthy lifestyle you deserve to live. Intentions to adjust your lifestyle are great, but intentions are just that until you have a plan. Planning out the adjustments will also help changing your life not feel like such a daunting task. Step-by-step, we will analyze and find practical ways to begin implementing a new way of living.

Weight management is the first step into changing your lifestyle. Whether you're overweight or underweight, both can be detrimental to your health and the function of your hormones. Being overweight can lead to constant high levels of insulin, called hyperinsulinemia. Unfortunately, this condition can cause short-term and long-term issues like extra weight gain, and eventually lead to serious medical issues like cancer or heart disease. You could also develop insulin resistance which causes your pancreas to produce even more insulin, creating a vicious cycle of insulin production (Healthline, 2021).

However, there are many steps to take to lower your insulin and manage your weight. Cutting out excess carbohydrates is one of the best ways to manage high insulin levels. Carbs raise your blood sugar and insulin levels more than proteins and healthy fats. There are many studies that have proven a low carb diet can lower insulin levels and increase insulin sensitivity, combating insulin resistance. Another great way to manage your weight is to watch your portion sizes. Overeating is one of the biggest reasons for high insulin levels because your pancreas has different amounts of insulin to help process different types and amounts of food. Lowering your overall intake of all forms of sugar can help you manage your weight struggles. Replacing processed sugar with natural types of sugar such as fruit, honey, and agave can help lower your insulin levels and weight. Of course, regular exercise needs to be implemented into your weekly routine.

Adding things like an apple cider vinegar shot after eating carbs and cinnamon into your food and drinks can also help you to manage your weight. Cinnamon is full of healthy antioxidants and according to Healthline, "Recent studies suggest that both individuals living with insulin resistance and those with relatively normal insulin levels who supplement with cinnamon may experience enhanced insulin levels and decreased insulin levels," (Healthline, 2021). Apple cider vinegar has been proven to lower insulin and blood glucose levels when taken after a heavy-carb meal. Two to six tablespoons of apple cider vinegar are recommended to lower insulin and blood sugar levels (Healthline, 2021).

Another big way to manage weight is through the leptin hormone. Being overweight can cause your leptin levels to become resistant. Remember, leptin is the hormone that tells your brain when you're full. If your leptin levels become resistant, your brain will not understand that you're full and this can cause overeating. A great way to combat this is staying on an anti-inflammatory diet, exercising, taking fish oil, and keeping a good sleep schedule. Ghrelin is another hormone that tells your brain when to stop eating. If these get out of balance, this can lead to overeating and weight gain. Some great ways to get the ghrelin levels back in balance are to avoid processed sugars and eat healthy lean proteins (Healthline, 2021).

Being underweight can impact your hormones negatively, as well. Being underweight can make it hard for your body to get adequate nutrients that it needs to support your hormones. The biggest issue which can arise from being underweight is issues with fertility and the reproductive system. For women, being underweight can cause your body to stop producing estrogen. When estrogen production stops, your body will stop ovulating and menstrual cycles will stop, as well. For men, being underweight can slow or stop the production of testosterone. Testosterone is what creates healthy sperm, so when this becomes imbalanced, fertility issues could become a concern. Getting on a steady diet full of healthy fats, lean proteins, and healthy carbohydrates can help balance this out. Also, cutting back or modifying your workouts can help you put on healthy weight (Columbia Fertility Associates, 2021).

The next step in changing our lifestyle is getting adequate sleep to support your body. Sleep plays an enormous role in balancing out hormones. While getting eight hours of sleep might sound like a fantasy world, inadequate sleep can have serious effects on your health and metabolism. According to an article from the Scientific American, "Research found that studies of people without sleep-related conditions who got consecutive nights of four to six hours of sleep revealed a wide range of negative side effects involving appetite hormone, signaling, physical activity, eating behavior, and even fat-loss rate," (Scientific American, 2021). This is because sleep deprivation can mess with the hunger signaling hormones, ghrelin, and leptin. It can also significantly decrease your amount of physical activity throughout the day. When your body is physically exhausted, it does not have the correct amount of energy stored in order to accomplish the high-intensity exercise. This can affect your metabolism and overall health.

Sleep deprivation can also lead to an increase in cortisol. And we know the effects of high cortisol can take a toll on our physical well-being, especially when it comes to weight gain. A recent study found that people who were sleep-deprived developed higher levels of cortisol later in the day, even though this is the time cortisol should be lowering as your body prepares for sleep. When cortisol is heightened during the time it should be lowering, your metabolism cannot process normally. This means that it will begin to store fat and use muscle as energy (Scientific American, 2021).

Okay, but how do we fix this problem? Let's start by dissecting what happens when we sleep. Sleep is divided into three stages, each ninety minutes long. Each stage is either a cycle of rapid eye movement or non-rapid eye movement sleep. These cycles repeat throughout the night, depending on how long we sleep. The first stage is referred to as N1, and it consists of light sleep, right in the beginning of the night when you first fall asleep. During N2, your body temperature drops and you are unaware of your surroundings. N3 is the most important stage of the sleep cycle as it's the deepest and when your body heals and restores energy. This stage is also where your hunger hormones are released (Hormone Health Network, 2019).

A disruption to any one of these cycles can be harmful to your hormones and health long-term. Most people think weekends are for "catching up on sleep," but in reality, sleeping in on weekends can make it more difficult to find and maintain a regular sleep schedule. A great first step into finding a sleep schedule is to change the time you eat dinner. If you consistently eat dinner late at night, your body will be awake longer trying to process the food. Avoiding snacking late at night is also important. Drinking a lot of caffeine, especially after lunchtime can also keep you awake longer. Minimizing cell phones, laptops or any electronic use can help you fall asleep faster. The light from the screens can wire your brain, sending confusing signals that it's time to wake up. Also, be sure to keep track of any disturbances you experience during the night. Did you have to get up a lot to use the bathroom? Did you wake up because something was hurting? Keeping track of these things and bringing them to your doctor can help you regulate your sleep schedule (Hormone Health Network, 2019).

The truth is that even a single night of sleep deprivation can tank our energy and mess with our metabolism. One night of sleep deprivation can also mess with our hunger hormones and create a small resistance leading into the next day. Chronic sleep deprivation can cause an irregular appetite, mess with your blood sugar levels, and put you at risk for diabetes. Overall, the risk of diabetes, insulin resistance, imbalanced levels of ghrelin and leptin, and obesity. Sleep is where our body does most of our inner work on our health, and not maintaining a healthy sleep schedule can lead to chronic hormone imbalances (Endocrinol, 2015).

The next great way to change your lifestyle is by doing yoga on a regular basis. It might seem strange, but yoga has numerous health benefits that can positively impact your hormones. When we think of our hormones, we now know that it is a complex system that is extremely sensitive to outside stimuli. However, there are some outside stimuli that can positively benefit our hormones, and one of those is yoga. First, there are many different practices of yoga, and specific ones can help keep the entire endocrine system in balance. Second, there are also specific poses that can affect and target specific glands to help regulate our hormones. This can create positive stimuli all over our body and help to bring back consistent production of certain hormones we might be lacking in. Another way yoga is fantastic for balancing out hormones is its focus on breathing. These breathing techniques can awaken the entire endocrine system. They can also bring back its primary functions while promoting stability. Yoga is great stress relief, as well. The over physical exertion combined with the meditative nature of yoga can bring our hormones and endocrine system back to homeostasis (Health Shots. 2021).

Let's take a look at some breathing techniques that are beneficial in balancing hormones and overall health. The first, known as the 4-7-8 technique, or pranayama, is designed to stimulate relaxation and bring stillness to the body. This technique can be specifically helpful in getting your digestion back on track. Because our body is able to handle digestion better when it is calm, chronic stress can hurt our digestion and nutrient intake. We want to get our bodies back to viewing digestion as a priority, and this is a great technique to achieve that. You can use this technique before a meal in order to help your body reach the state of relaxation needed for proper digestion. You can also use this technique if you are still feeling stress is messing with your appetite and stomach.

Here are the steps of the 4-7-8 technique: "Begin in either a sitting position or laying down, and then exhale through your mouth making a whooshing sound. Next, close your mouth and inhale through your nose while silently counting to four. Following this, hold your breath for seven seconds. Then repeat the first step by making a whooshing exhale through your mouth for eight seconds. Repeat the process at least four times, working your way up to eight cycles," (Boston Functional Nutrition, 2021).

Another great technique for hormone balance is the "alternate nostril breathing" technique. This greatly benefits your melatonin levels and helps bring peace to your mind to help you fall asleep faster. It is great for lowering anxiety and improving your metabolism as well as respiratory and cognitive functions. It's believed to help clear negative energy and promote healthy serotonin levels, and bring cortisol back under control (Boston Function Nutritional, 2021).

Here are the steps to practice this technique: "Begin by sitting comfortably with your legs crossed. Next, exhale completely and then use your right thumb to close your right nostril. Inhale through your left nostril, then before exhaling, close off the left nostril with your fingers. Remove your thumb from the right nostril and exhale through the right side. Inhale through the right side, then close off this nostril. Exhale through the left nostril and inhale, then switch sides before exhaling again. You can do this as many times as you want, but always finish by exhaling on the left side," (Boston Functional Nutrition, 2021).

Now, let's look at some yoga poses that are fantastic for balancing hormone health. The first one we are going to talk about is commonly known as the Cobra Pose but is also referred to as "bhujangasana." Cobra Pose can help to stimulate your adrenal gland, thereby allowing your system to handle stress better and also release some pent-up tension. "To do this pose, you will start by lying flat on your stomach with your legs together and your palms flat on the floor beside your shoulders. Your head will start resting flat on the floor, and you can then lift your head and chest upward. Hold this pose for up to a minute, inhaling and exhaling deeply, before lowering yourself back down toward the ground. Repeat this pose a few times to really enjoy the benefits," Mind Body Green, 2021).

Another great pose known as the Rabbit Pose or, Sasangasana, helps with hormone balance by activating your thyroid glands. This can help fight depression and promote healthy calcium regulation to our systems. "To begin, start by sitting on your knees on your mat. Extend your arms back and hold onto the soles of your feet. Tuck your chin inward toward your chest as you round your body forward, hinging your body at your hips. Your head should drop toward the floor as your forehead touches your knees. Lift your hips upward slightly as the crown of your head rests on the floor, and rest comfortably for five deep breaths," (Mind Body Green, 2021).

We know that stress can be one of the most detrimental factors affecting our hormones. To recap, stress can cause a variety of symptoms from nights sweats, sleep disturbances, anxiety, low sex drive, and leg cramps. Chronic stress can also leave us feeling isolated and low in our self-worth. Dr. Jane Oh stated, "Americans are living life at 100 miles per hour, every day. It's no wonder we have hormonal imbalances. When patients come to me for hormonal imbalance, the root cause is usually too much cortisol or stress hormone. Then it's a downstream- every other hormone in our bodies is affected, including sex hormones and thyroid," (Healthline, 2021).

Since most of us are under relentless stress in our day-to-day lives, another lifestyle change we must learn is stress management. That might seem like a broad view of a large task, however, there are plenty of small, practical ways to manage our stress. The first step is to identify the reasons behind your stress and face them head-on. Recognizing the cause of your stress and saying it out loud has a way to make the stress not seem so gigantic or overwhelming. Once you have identified it, you can begin to actively combat it and lower your stress.

Learning how to remain calm during adverse and stressful times can bring regulation to our endocrine system. Some other great ways to reduce stress are the daily habits you adjust and adapt. Practicing meditation and breathing techniques on a daily basis, maintaining a regular exercise routine, minimizing the amount of caffeine and alcohol you consume, practicing a healthy diet, and re-working your work-life balance are some practical ways to manage your stress levels (Healthline, 2021).

The last lifestyle change we are going to address is intermittent fasting. This is a fairly new diet trend that has been praised for its numerous health benefits including hormonal health. However, we are going to take a closer look at intermittent fasting, because everyone is different and this approach to nutrition might not work for some. Intermittent fasting is a pattern of eating that cycles between times of eating and times of fasting. For intermittent fasting, it doesn't focus on what you eat as much as it focuses on when you eat. Now, this can be problematic considering a healthy diet is vital for our overall health, but intermittent fasting with the correct diet can be beneficial for balancing your hormones. This is due to the fact that when you are fasting, your insulin levels begin to drop. Your fat eventually begins to burn away because the longer time between meals, the more your insulin supply is exhausted (SCL Health, 2021).

According to James Roche, a registered dietitian nutritionist, "Intermittent fasting could take place in any specific period of time, although 8/16, eight hours for eating and sixteen hours for fasting, or 10/14, ten hours for eating and fourteen for fasting, are the two most common approaches. It is recommended the starting time be earlier in the day to optimize metabolism and avoid eating at the end of the day or late at night, which is linked to increased fat storage and inefficient use of food," (SCL Health, 2021).

So, what can intermittent fasting do for your hormones? First, it can lower your overall inflammation which we know is a great way to balance your hormones. Second, it can lower oxidative stress and blood sugar levels. It can also help neurons grow and increase serotonin, which is effective in fighting depression. Last, it can help our metabolism function when we sleep, which can bring back energy and burn more calories. These are all amazing benefits that can come with intermittent fasting. However, it is important to remember that the things we eat do have the ability to positively or negatively impact our health. Choosing this route is a great way to change your lifestyle, but please remember to eat the correct foods for your hormones and health while intermittent fasting (SCL Health, 2021).

Life can be difficult, stressful, and overwhelming. All of these things and more can lead to health issues, including hormonal imbalances. However, these lifestyle changes can change the course of your health and hormones. Too often, as the years go by, we find ourselves simply surviving the day-to-day. But it isn't enough to just survive. Stress does not mean you have to stop living. Taking care of yourself and your hormones is just as important as taking care of your family, career, or relationships. So often, our focus shifts and we tend to neglect ourselves. But nothing can thrive if you aren't. Remembering that you are just as important as everything else in your life is the key to reclaiming your health! Because if you're not healthy and happy, then nothing else will be either.

Chapter Summary

- Weight management for being either over or underweight is vital for our hormonal health and there are many great ways to achieve this.
- Managing your sleep schedule is a great way to balance your hormones because lack of sleep can be detrimental to your health.
- Yoga is a great manager of stress and hormones.
- Intermittent fasting is not just a fad, but maintaining the proper diet while doing it is key.

In the next chapter, you will learn....

- The importance of having a plan for your meals.
- How to stick to this plan and change your mindset around food.
- What a day-to-day plan looks like and the ways you can make it easy.

PLAN MY LIFE
MEAL PLANNING FOR
HORMONAL IMBALANCE

"Only when you identify and accept your weaknesses will you finally stop running from your past." -David Goggins

If you have made it this far, then thank you and congratulations! We have arrived at the last chapter and final part of regaining our hormonal health through natural ways. In this last section, we are going to look at how establishing a good meal plan can change our hormones and bring them back to balance. We will also compare it with what an incorrect meal plan looks like and discuss the differences proper eating can make in our overall health. When we think of meal planning, most of us equate it to hardcore gymgoers who meal prep every second of their lives. However, this isn't necessarily the case. Meal planning is knowing what you are going to be eating in the upcoming days and how those foods affect your body.

Right about now, you might be wondering why you need a meal plan. If you know the right foods, why do you need a detailed plan to go with them? Because staying consistent at changing your life and diet is impossible if you're not willing to face your bad habits, and set a plan in place to remedy them. Having a tangible, visual plan will hold you accountable for staying consistent at the work you're about to put into it. Facing your own bad habits also makes them real and easier to overcome. This isn't about being mean to yourself, but saying your bad habits out loud, makes it real, and makes the changes you are about to implement real as well! Everyone wants results, but most forget that real results only come from consistent, hard work over an extended period of time. There is no magic pill, no fast-track way to get there. You must be willing to put in the work, time and dedication it takes to change your life. Having a meal plan in place makes it easier and less overwhelming to stick to that plan.

Let's recap some of the foods that are great for our hormones. Flaxseed, wild salmon, broccoli, lentils, sunflower seeds, and sweet potatoes are all great foods for balancing your sex hormones. These include progesterone, estrogen, and testosterone. The above foods contain high levels of vitamin D. This is great for the production and secretion of sex hormones. Omega-3 fatty acids, lean proteins, and fiber help remove excess estrogen from our systems. All of these factors are beneficial to our natural hormone production and balance (Academy of Culinary Nutrition, 2021).

For our thyroid hormones, foods like seaweed, brazil nuts, sardines, spinach, and quinoa are fantastic. They contain iodine. This is a mineral that helps our thyroid hormone function properly. Additionally, they contain antioxidants and selenium. These protect your thyroid gland, vitamin B12, and zinc (Academy of Culinary Nutrition, 2021).

Some foods good for our adrenal glands include bell peppers, kale, avocado, pumpkin seeds, almonds, sea salt, eggs, and millet. Even though bell peppers are a nightshade, they also contain high amounts of vitamin C. This is an essential vitamin to help our adrenals function. Kale also contains high levels of vitamins C, K, and A. Avocado and almonds are both fantastic sources of healthy fats. They help maintain regular blood sugar levels. Eggs are beneficial because they contain omega-3 fatty acids. Millet is a great gluten free form of whole grain. Sea salt replaces sodium levels and keeps us from developing salt cravings (Academy of Culinary Nutrition, 2021).

Now, before we begin the plans of a good meal plan, let's outline what a bad one would look like and why. Let's say you've prepped your meal plan and decided that large amounts of protein and higher carb intake is the route you want to go. If you're suffering from hormone imbalance, this might not be the route for you. Let's say your meal prep for the next five days includes protein pancakes for breakfast, salads for lunch, and red meat with carbs for dinner. That doesn't sound bad right? Well, let's take a look. You begin your day with a large cup of coffee, milk, and protein pancakes. For lunch, you have a salad with cheese, lots of different peppers, chicken, and ranch. For dinner, you plan to have a large piece of red meat, and pasta. This is not the ideal diet plan if you want to manage your hormonal imbalance.

Beginning your day with milk, heavy amounts of protein can shift your hormone production. Milk leads to inflammation and can disrupt the microbiome in your gut. Too much caffeine can stress out your body and cause your cortisol levels to increase and heavy amounts of protein first thing in the morning can be too harsh for your stomach to digest. When we think about breakfast, we often think it's the most important meal of the day, because this is what we've been taught. However, this isn't necessarily true. While it is important to begin your day with good nutrients, it's equally as important to listen to our bodies, as well. Some people's stomachs wake up later than others, so don't force yourself to eat first thing in the morning if you aren't hungry. Eat a good source of nutrients when you begin to feel hungry because that means your stomach is ready and able to digest food (Health Shots, 2021).

While everyone equates salads with healthy eating, it is easy to use them in incorrect ways. Covering a salad in dairy, harsh vegetables, and processed protein is a sure-fire way to hurt your hormones. While vegetables such as peppers, tomatoes, potatoes, and kale have great health benefits, if they are consumed in excess, they can cause a thyroid imbalance and cause inflammation. Limiting these vegetables, dairy intake, and finding a healthy fat to throw in is a much better lunch for our diet plan (Health Shots, 2021).

While protein and carbs are promoted as good sources of energy, for someone struggling with hormonal imbalance, they can be detrimental. Red meat can increase estrogen production and is full of saturated fat. Heavy carbs are sure to hurt your stomach and digestion process, meaning your body won't have time or room for anything else. Instead, we need to find great alternate sources of protein, carbs, and always include a serving of nutrient-rich vegetables (Health Shots, 2021).

So, what does a good meal plan look like? We are going to take a look at some great examples and various ideas of amazing meal plans that will help you start your health journey off right. We are going to start small, with a meal plan for three days, working our way up to meal planning for the entire week. Having a plan for the foods to eat to nurture our body can make the process less overwhelming. Completely changing the way, we think about food and our entire diet can seem impossible as a whole. But, breaking it down step by step, we will learn that it's not as daunting of a task as it might seem.

Let's start with a three-day plan to get our systems back on track. To begin the day, we don't need to start nutrient-rich with a large plate of food to give us energy. This information is simply false. When you first wake up, drinking something with a good source of acid in it can be extremely beneficial to your digestive system. Dr. Jonathan V. Wright says, "When we carefully test people over the age of forty who are having heartburn, indigestion, and gas, over ninety percent of the time we find inadequate acid production by the stomach," (Mind Body Green, 2021). However, you don't have to be suffering from heartburn for your body to need this. Preparing our body for food intake for the rest of the day is vital. Diluting two tablespoons of apple cider vinegar in eight ounces of water with some lemon added is a great way to achieve this (Mind Body Green, 2021).

When your body is ready for breakfast, make sure it is a healthy source of fiber with a little bit of protein. It will boost your energy levels for the rest of the day. It should not contain high amounts of sugar or carbs. These can leave you feeling jittery for the rest of the day. Some great examples of great breakfast choices include eggs, chia seeds, nuts, avocado, grass-fed butter, and coconut oil, and any kind of vegetable (Mind Body Green, 2021). An easy way to achieve this is to use your morning coffee as a way to gain nutrients for the day. One cup of coffee is okay, and adding half a tablespoon of coconut oil and a little bit of unsalted butter can give you a great energy source. It might sound crazy, but first, adding these to your coffee and blending it up tastes like a delicious latte. Second, beginning your day with healthy fats boosts your metabolism and gives you a reserve for energy.

If you are a person who runs on caffeine, this can be detrimental to your hormones, as well. Instead of running for that midday cup of coffee, try switching it out with tea. Coffee can stress out the adrenals and acids in your stomach. Teas like green tea, ginger tea, and tulsi tea can be super beneficial for your hormones as well as a great replacement for coffee. All of these teas also replenish your adrenal glands and boost energy levels, as well. You can find all of these teas at your local health food store and sometimes grocery store as well (Mind Body Green, 2021).

Now, a salad is always a good idea for lunch, as long as we are adding the right ingredients. First of all, while a sandwich might sound healthy, it contains gluten and dairy which cause inflammation. Staying away from both of these products is very important if we want to balance our hormones. Instead, a salad with lots of cruciferous vegetables can be helpful to our liver and thyroid. Adding arugula, kale, cabbage, or broccoli to a will give you the correct nutrients you need. Also adding a lean source of protein such as free-range chicken, wild salmon, or grass-fed beef can give you the right protein for the rest of your day. Next, we want to add some color to that salad, and beets or carrots are both fantastic for hormone health. They help to detox our system and make room for new hormones. The dressing you add should contain extra-virgin olive oil, citrus, and some vinegar. Add a little bit of salt and a spice, and you have a delicious lunch (Mind Body Green, 2021).

Dinner should never be a feast. We live in a culture that promotes dinner as a time to eat our largest meal of the day, however, this makes it difficult for our stomach to eat the food. First, dinner should never be super late and we need to make sure we are not eating heavy or hard things to process. This can mess with everything from our sleep pattern to metabolic process. A great and easy thing to plan is soups. Soups and stews can last all week, and also contain the perfect balance of nutrients you need. Be sure not to add thickeners like wheat flour as that causes inflammation in our body. If soup isn't your thing, try a lean source of protein like fish, a low-carb food like rice, and a green vegetable like broccoli (Mind Body Green, 2021).

Now, let's look at what a realistic meal plan looks like for an entire week. Again, every morning you should begin with apple cider vinegar. It's affordable and can be found in your local grocery store. This will set your stomach acids at a good level for the rest of your day.

Day 1: When your stomach is awake and ready, make a cup of coffee with coconut oil and butter and then have a breakfast that includes lean protein and fiber. Toasted gluten-free or organic grain bread with an egg and avocado is a great place to start. For a snack drink some green tea and eat some almonds. For lunch, a bowl with cauliflower rice, a cruciferous vegetable, and a lean source of protein is ideal. For dinner, lettuce wraps with free-range chicken and some peppers and zucchini is a great way to keep it nice and light. End the day with a cup of chamomile tea to help your body relax (Rocky Mountain Analytical, 2021).

Day 2: A great, sustainable breakfast is quinoa-based oatmeal topped with berries, nuts, and raw honey. For a snack, drink some ginger tea to reset your digestion and eat some slices of apple for natural sugar. For lunch, a spinach-based salad with carrots, tomatoes, and a homemade olive oil dressing is perfect. A great dinner idea is a healthy version of pasta. This is spaghetti squash, with a lean protein like ground turkey (Rocky Mountain Analytical, 2021).

Day 3: Another great breakfast consists of sauteing sweet potato hash with some peppers, a green vegetable, onions, and garlic. Add an egg on top for protein! For a healthy snack, grab some carrots, bell peppers, and hummus for something filling but light. For lunch, try a healthy stir fry bowl. Include lots of veggies like snap peas, carrots, and broccoli. Top it with a lean protein like chicken or salmon. If you're missing burgers, substitute it with a lean turkey patty in a lettuce wrap. Add toppings like avocado, tomatoes, and your favorite sugar-free condiment (Rocky Mountain Analytical, 2021).

Day 4: Keeping it simple, breakfast consists of a bulletproof coffee (unsalted butter and coconut oil blended) and mixed berries, and an egg. For a midday snack, drink a cup of green tea and have some macadamia nuts. They are full of healthy fat and will keep your energy going for longer!

For lunch, create a salad with shrimp, cruciferous vegetables, pecans, and your homemade olive oil dressing. For dinner, use the oven to bake chicken wings with olive oil, salt, and pepper (Rocky Mountain Analytical, 2021).

Day 5: After your daily apple cider vinegar routine, have chia seed pudding or an açai bowl. These are full of antioxidants and will keep you feeling full and energetic. For a snack, grab a handful of almonds and some dark, organic chocolate. Dark chocolate is a great way to satisfy your sweet tooth without the added sugar. For lunch, try making some gluten-free pasta salad. Add lots of veggies like spinach, mushrooms, and bell peppers. Use a homemade olive oil dressing. Add some range-free chicken if you feel like you need the protein. Before dinner, drink a cup of green, ginger, or peppermint tea to settle your digestion. For dinner, cook a lean, grass-fed steak. Add roasted or grilled green beans with mushrooms and onions. Finish with some roasted, organic red potatoes (Rocky Mountain Analytical, 2021).

Okay! Now that you have a solid base for a five-day meal plan, you can begin to expand from there. There are so many great options for eating healthy and balancing your hormones. Beginning your day with nutrient-rich sustaining foods is the best way to make sure your energy doesn't dip too low before lunch. One to two snacks a day that is full of healthy fats will help your cravings for all that unhealthy junk to disappear. Kicking your midday coffee habit will settle your adrenals and thyroid. Making sure your lunch is well balanced will stop the "food coma" that should never happen. And not eating too late and keeping it light will help support your metabolic process!

Before we bring this last chapter to a close, we need to look at how we prepare food and the correlation it has to our hormones. See, the way we prepare our food can make a world of difference in its nutritional value. Baking or stove cooking your proteins rather than frying them is important to balance out hormones. Fried foods are simply not good for the metabolic process or your thyroid hormones. The cleaner and easier the preparation, the healthier it probably is. Avoid thickening sauces with full-fat dairy products and try using milk substitutes instead. Artificial sweeteners aside from stevia, honey, and agave should be avoided as well. The ingredients you use to cook with are important too! You should avoid using vegetable and peanut oil. Unfortunately, these oils contain artificial fillers and cause a mess with the balance of your hormones. Instead, use products like coconut and olive oil, as well as organic butter. These are healthy fats that are honest in their ingredients.

As you learn and grow through this process, you will begin to adapt and develop your recipes and meals which work with your body. We are all different, but the truth is that food is either the making or undoing of our health. Trust the process, this guide, but most importantly, yourself. You have all the information necessary to make the best change in your life, starting today. Start by changing the way you think about food. Remember, food is not a form of entertainment, it is a source of energy, and our bodies will respond to whatever kind of energy we put into it. There is no substitute for hard work and dedication. With a little guidance and preparation, you can change your hormonal health. There is more to life than simply surviving the day-to-day. Love yourself enough to start living again.

Chapter Summary

- Having a plan is important because change doesn't come with hard work, but having a guideline makes that work less overwhelming.

- A bad meal plan can affect your hormones in many different ways, so it's important to know the meal plans to avoid.

- Using a basic guide for a five-day meal plan can help you begin to develop your own.

- Food is not a source of entertainment, but rather, a source of energy.

FINAL WORDS

"Don't wait. The time will never be just right." -Napoleon Hill

After reading this book there are a few things I hope you have accomplished. I hope you have a new understanding of your hormones, their functions, and why they can so easily become imbalanced. I hope you have a deeper knowledge of the different types of imbalances and how they can affect your body. I hope you have a new sense of hope in gaining your health back naturally. And finally, I hope you feel confident to push forward and make the dietary and life changes necessary to achieve hormonal balance.

I also hope you feel more in tune with your body and hormones. I hope you have realized your body is never against you, but rather, always trying to work for you. It sometimes gets confused and over or under produces things in an attempt to protect you. But your body loves you! It's constantly fighting to maintain homeostasis so you can live a healthy life. Your body deserves the same love it shows you.

Our bodies are made up of a complex system.

Hormones play a huge role in maintaining the inner workings of that system. There are so many different kinds of imbalances. It can be easy for your hormones to become unbalanced. This does not mean it's impossible to bring your body back to the center. There is much more hope for hormone imbalances than having to get on a type of hormone replacement or surgery. There are so many natural ways to change your hormones. Most of them provide fuel.

Supplements are a great place to start. Contact an expert. Get bloodwork to know which ones to take for your hormonal imbalance. There are so many different types and numerous areas that can be affected. Do not self-diagnose. Learn about the ingredients of these supplements and how they work to balance your hormones.

I hope you feel more comfortable with working out. Not everyone has to live in the gym to become healthy. Your physical activity should include things you genuinely enjoy, that way it'll be easier to maintain. Working out should be more than just a task you must accomplish, it should be a hobby! It takes a mindset change, but when you shift your focus, it will make all the difference.

I hope you feel less intimidated by the concept of eating healthy. We live in a world where new diets are a regular occurrence, and everyone believes they have the key to our overall health. The truth is, there is no magic pill or fast track to getting your hormones and health back in order. Food is nutrients and nothing more. It's as simple and complicated as that. Understanding the properties of what we are putting into our bodies is essential for understanding what drives it. This is the way you begin to change your life.

More than anything, I hope you believe in your ability to take control of your health. Changing your life is just about changing your mindset around food or exercise. It's about changing the way you think and what you believe about yourself. If you believe you can or if you believe you cannot, you're probably right. We spend most of our lives wishing for a better body, health, or brain. Whatever you want, know that you are enough in yourself. The only reason you want this change is that you deserve to live a healthy and vibrant life. Believe that you can do this because you deserve this! Altering your eating habits and physical activity is less challenging when you take the right steps.

There will never be a perfect time to begin something new. Making major life changes will never be easy. Life will always throw curve balls and unforeseen circumstances your way. So, stop. waiting for the right time to change your diet, habits, and. routines. You deserve the same time, love, and care you give to everything else. Now, you are equipped with all the tools necessary to make those changes! The time to reclaim your health and life is now. Start choosing yourself, today and every day that follows. And if you enjoyed this book, give it a little love on Amazon too.

REFERENCES

Biggers, Alana., Osborn, Corinne. 2020. "Everything You Should Know About Hormonal Imbalance." Healthline. Updated October 31, 2020.
https://www.healthline.com/health/hormonal-imbalance.

Chapel Hill Gynecology. 2019. "7 Lifestyle Habits that Can Affect Your Hormones."
https://chapelhillgynecology.com/lifestyle-habits-that-can-affect-your-hormones/.

Cleveland Clinic. 2019. "What's the Deal with Nightshade Vegetables?"
https://health.clevelandclinic.org/whats-the-deal-with-nightshade-vegetables/.

Cleveland Clinic. 2020. "Birth Control: The Pill."
https://my.clevelandclinic.org/health/drugs/3977-birth-control-the-pill.

Columbia Fertility Associates. 2021. "How Being Underweight or Overweight Can Affect Your Fertility." Accessed October 2, 2021.
https:// www.columbiafertility.com/blog/how-being- underweight-or-overweight-can-affect-your-fertility.

Complete Care. 2021. "11 Best Supplements for Balancing Women's Hormones." Accessed September 20, 2021.
https://completecare.net/11-supplements-naturally-balance- hormones/.

Coyle Institute. 2021. "Teenage Hormone Imbalance: When to Talk to a Doctor." Accessed September 23, 2021.
https://coyleinstitute.com/understanding-teenage-hormone- imbalance/.

Desai, Jag. 2019. "Male Hormone Imbalance: What You Should Know." Core Medical & Wellness.
https://coremedicalwellness.com/male-hormone-imbalance-what-you-should-know/.

Duly Health Care. 2021. "5 Hormone Imbalances to Be Aware Of." Accessed September 24, 2021.
https://www.dulyhealthandcare.com/health-topic/five-hormone-imbalances-to-be- aware- of.

Elist, James. 2020. "Drinking Water and Hormonal Balance." Dr. Elist MD Facts.
https:// www.drelist.com/blog/drinking-water-hormonal-balance/.

Ecklekamp, Stephanie. 2019. "10 Signs You Have a Hormonal Imbalance." Parsley Health. Updated July 15, 2019.
https://www.parsleyhealth.com/blog/hormonal-imbalance-symptoms/.

Ernst, Holly., Huizen, Jennifer. 2020. "What to Know About Hormonal Imbalances." Medical News Today.
https://www.medicalnewstoday.com/articles/321486.

Food Empowerment Project. 2021. "Fast Food." Accessed September 20, 2021.
https:// foodispower.org/access-health/fast-food/.

Geetika, Sachdev. 2020. "What's Healthier: Suji or Whole Wheat? Let's Settle the Debate Once and for All." Health Shots.
https://www.healthshots.com/healthy-eating/nutrition/whats-healthier-suji-or-whole-wheat/amp.

Gottfried, Sara. 2021. "The 10 Best Types of Protein for Hormone Balance." Mind Body Green. Updated January 4, 2021.
https://amp.mindbodygreen.com/articles/how-protein-affects-your-hormones.

Happy Hormones for Life. 2020. "Why Healthy Fats are so Good for Your Hormones."
https://happyhormonesforlife.com/healthy-fats/.

Harmon, Katherine. 2012. "How Slight Sleep Deprivation Could Add Extra Pounds." Scientific American.
https://www.scientificamerican.com/article/sleep-deprivation-obesity/.

Harvard Health. 2020. "Exercising to Relax: How Does Exercise Reduce Stress? Surprising Answers to this Question and More."
https://www.health.harvard.edu/staying-healthy/exercising-to-relax.

HWC. 2021. "Hormone Diet Plan." Accessed October 2, 2021.
https://hwcoftexas.com/wp-content/uploads/2015/10/HormoneDietPlan.pdf.

Jefferson Health. 2019. "The Other Side of Anaerobic Exercise: How the Human Growth Hormone Helps All Ages."

https://newjersey.jeffersonhealth.org/content/ot her-side-anaerobic-exercise-how-human- growth-hormone-helps-all-ages.

Khalfan, Ferwa. 2021. "Nutrition + Diet for Women's Hormone Balance, Fertility + Postpartum." Aristos. Accessed September 30, 2021.
https://www.aristoslifestyle.com/articles/nutritio n-diet-for-womens-fertility-hormones-postpartum.

Krivoshen, Jennifer. 2021. "Balancing Hormones with Food." Rocky Mountain Analytical. Accessed October 1, 2021.
https://rmalab.com/balancing-hormones-with-food/.

Lawrenson, Amy. 2021. "This is How to Help Balance Your Hormones with Exercise,   According to Experts." Byrdie. Updated August 9, 2021.
https://www.byrdie.com/exercise-to-balance-hormones.

Martinez, Ramon., Ruiz, Daniel. 2019. "Sleep and Circadian Rhythm." Hormone Health Network. Updated June, 2019.
https://www.hormone.org/your-health-and-hormones/sleep-and-circadian-rhythm.

Mayo Clinic Staff. 2020. "Testosterone Therapy: Potential Benefits and Risks as You Age." Mayo Clinic.
https://www.mayoclinic.org/healthy-lifestyle/sexual-health/in-depth/testosterone- therapy/art-20045728.

McMillen, Matt. 2019. "Testosterone Replacement Therapy: Myths and Facts." WebMD.

https://www.webmd.com/men/replacement-therapy.

Medanta. 2019. "Surgery for Hyperthyroidism: Are You a Candidate for a Thyroid Gland Removal?" https://www.medanta.org/patient-education-blog/surgery-for-hyperthyroidism-are-you-a- candidate-for-a-thyroid-gland-removal/.

Merck Manual. 2021. "Effects of Aging on the Endocrine System." Accessed September 27, 2021. https://www.merckmanuals.com/home/hormon al-and-metabolic-disorders/biology-of-the-endocrine-system/effects-of-aging-on-the-endocrine-system.

Montagu, Julie., Talebian, Sheeva. 2020. "3 Easy Yoga Poses To Balance Out-Of-Whack Hormones." Mind Body Green. Updated January 15, 2020. https://amp.mindbodygreen.com/articles/3-easy-yoga-poses-to-balance-out-of-whack-hormones--25333.

Moody, Liz., Talebian, Sheeva. 2019. "These 8 Foods Are Wreaking Havoc on Your Hormones." Mind Body Green. Updated 7, 2019. https://www.mindbodygreen.com/0-29200/these-8-foods-are-wreaking-havoc-on-your-hormones.html.

Moody Month. 2021. "How do Vitamins Affect Your Hormones and Mood?" https://moodymonth.com/articles/how-do-vitamins-affect-your-hormones-and-mood.

National Cancer Institute. 2021. "Characteristics of Hormones." Accessed September 15, 2021. https://training.seer.cancer.gov/anatomy/endocri

ne/hormones.html.

Northrop, Alyssa., Spritzler, Franziska. 2021. "14 Ways to Lower Your Insulin Levels." Healthline.
https://www.healthline.com/nutrition/14-ways-to-lower-insulin.

OB/GYN Associates of America. 2021. "Hormones and Weight Gain: How to Fix the Hormones That control Your Weight." Accessed October 1, 2021.
https://obgynal.com/hormones-and-weight-gain/.

Osteopathic Center for Healing. 2021. "Signs and Symptoms of Male Hormone Imbalance." Accessed September 20, 2021.
https://www.drneilspiegel.com/blog/signs-and-symptoms-of-male-hormone-imbalance.

Pagán, Camille. 2021. "The Hormone Diet." Nourish by WebMD.
https://www.webmd.com/diet/a-z/hormone-diet.

Perry, Shannon. 2021. "Menopause and Dehydration: Drink More Water." Gennev. Updated August 30, 2021.
https://gennev.com/education/menopause-and-dehydration.

Peternell, Tracy. 2020. "Breaking Hormone Myths." Delicious Living.
https://www.deliciousliving.com/health/breaking-hormone-myths/.

Piedmont Healthcare. 2021. "How Exercise Helps Balance Hormones." Accessed September 28, 2021.
https://www.piedmont.org/living-better/how-

exercise-helps-balance-hormones.

O'Sullivan, Sadhbh. 2020. "Do You Really Need Those Insta-Friendly Supplements to Balance Your Hormones." Refinery29.
https://www.refinery29.com/amp/en-gb/hormone-balance-pills-do-they-work.

Rojas, Carol. 2020. "Can Stress Upset My Hormones?" Winnie Palmer Hospital.
https://www.winniepalmerhospital.com/content-hub/can-stress-upset-my-hormones.

Rush. 2021. "Hormones as You Age." Accessed September 29, 2021.
https://www.rush.edu/news/hormones-you-age.

SCL Health. 2021. "Does Intermittent Fasting Actually Work?" Accessed October 2, 2021.
https://www.sclhealth.org/blog/2021/04/does-intermittent-fasting-actually-work/.

Sethi, Shreya. 2021. "Try These 5 Yoga Asanas to Regulate Hormones and Enjoy Good Health." Health Shots.
https://www.healthshots.com/fitness/staying-fit/try-these-5-yoga-asanas-to-regulate-hormones-and-enjoy-good-health/amp.

Sharp, Abbey. 2018. "The Foods That Balance Out or Mess With) Your Hormones." Greatist.
https://greatist.com/eat/foods-for-hormonal-imbalance#1.

Snyder, Kristy. 2019. "How Long Does It Take to. Adjust to A New Birth Control Pill?" Nurx.
https://www.nurx.com/blog/how-long-does-it-

take-to-adjust-to-new-birth-control-pill/.

Spritzler, Franziska. 2017. "12 Natural Ways to Balance Your Hormones." Healthline.
https://www.healthline.com/nutrition/balance-hormones.

Stonewater Adolescent Recovery Center. 2020. "3 Ways Hormones Impact Teen Mental Health."
https://www.stonewaterrecovery.com/adolescent-treatment-blog/3-ways-hormones-impact-teen-mental-health/.

Talida. 2021. "5 Common Root Causes of Hormonal Imbalance." Hazel and Cacao.
https://hazelandcacao.com/5-common-root-causes-of-hormonal-imbalance/.

University Hospitals. 2021. "Comprehensive, Compassionate Care for Adolescent and Child Development." Accessed September 23, 2021.
https://www.uhhospitals.org/rainbow/services/pediatric-endocrinology/conditions-and-treatments/adolescent-hormonal-issues.

Wszelaki, Magdalena. 2019. "This. 3-Day Diet Will Balance Your Hormones, Stabilize Your Blood Sugar & Optimize Your Digestion." Mind Body Green. Updated October 7, 2019.
https://amp.mindbodygreen.com/articles/3-day-hormone-balance-diet-recipes-tips-tricks.

You and Your Hormones. 2021. "Endocrine Conditions." Accessed September 17, 2021.
https://www.yourhormones.info/endocrine-conditions/.

Younkin, Lainey. 2020. "Hormone-Balancing Foods: How Your Diet Can Help Keep Your Hormones Functioning Well." Eating Well.
https://www.eatingwell.com/article/7805452/hormone-balancing-foods-how-diet-can-help/.

Zorfass, Nina. 2020. "The Myths and Realities of Hormonal Imbalance (and Why Bio-   Individuality is Key)." Integrative Nutrition. Updated February 1, 2021.
https://www.integrativenutrition.com/blog/the-myths-and-realities-of-hormonal-   imbalance-and-why-bio-individuality-is-key

85026882R00090